Winter's End

Winter's End

Dementia and Dying Well

LEWIS COHEN, MD

Professor of Psychiatry Emeritus, Tufts University School
of Medicine, Boston, MA

and

Professor of Psychiatry Emeritus, University of Massachusetts
Chan School of Medicine, Worcester, MA

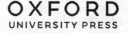

OXFORD
UNIVERSITY PRESS

OXFORD
UNIVERSITY PRESS

Oxford University Press is a department of the University of Oxford. It furthers
the University's objective of excellence in research, scholarship, and education
by publishing worldwide. Oxford is a registered trade mark of Oxford University
Press in the UK and certain other countries.

Published in the United States of America by Oxford University Press
198 Madison Avenue, New York, NY 10016, United States of America.

Library of Congress Cataloging-in-Publication Data
Names: Cohen, Lewis, author.
Title: Winter's end : dementia and dying well / Lewis Cohen.
Description: New York : Oxford University Press, [2024] |
Includes bibliographical references and index.
Identifiers: LCCN 2024006320 (print) | LCCN 2024006321 (ebook) |
ISBN 9780197748640 (paperback) | ISBN 9780197748664 (epub) |
ISBN 9780197748671
Subjects: MESH: Alzheimer Disease—psychology | Right to Die |
Attitude to Death | Interview
Classification: LCC RC523 (print) | LCC RC523 (ebook) | NLM WT 161 |
DDC 616.8/3110019—dc23/eng/20240327
LC record available at https://lccn.loc.gov/2024006320
LC ebook record available at https://lccn.loc.gov/2024006321

DOI: 10.1093/med/9780197748640.001.0001

Printed in Canada by Marquis Book Printing

The manufacturer's authorised representative in the EU for product safety is Oxford
University Press España S.A. of El Parque Empresarial San Fernando de Henares, Avenida
de Castilla, 2 – 28830 Madrid (www.oup.es/en or product.safety@oup.com). OUP España
S.A. also acts as importer into Spain of products made by the manufacturer.

In the service for the dead, the Catholic Church asks God to grant us all eternal rest. There is little fuss about Heaven or its glories. No fuss at all about Hell. Just eternal rest. And, after all the words squandered on right and wrong, failure and desire, love and the tragic failure to love, I am ready for eternal rest.

Eternal rest. Even the sound is soothing.

—John L'Heureux, His last essay, "On death and dignity," published in *The New Yorker Magazine*, April 29, 2019, before he received assisted dying for Parkinson's disease.

I can live with the fact that he decided thus, because he left us as a great glowing star, right on time, just before he would have collapsed into a stellar black hole.

—Guy Verhofstadt, Eulogy for celebrated Belgian author and poet, Hugo Claus, who had a dementia and was euthanized by his physician, from Wikipedia.

As far as my death is concerned, I feel strongly that I want to be held, I want to be sung to, and I want all the care hospice can provide. I want to be participatory in my end-of-life process. I get to choose how I'm going to die.

—Cheryl Hauser, Interview with Compassion and Choices, who had early-onset Alzheimer's disease and died after voluntarily stopping eating and drinking.

Knowing it to be inevitable, why not choose an aristocrat's death, ending life in a secret flourish, squandering any years that might have been? To die before coming to the end of willpower, was that not an aristocrat's choice?

—Frank Herbert, *Dune Messiah*, 1969

CONTENTS

INTRODUCTION

Seventy seemed to me to be a perfectly acceptable age to hang up my white coat and retire. I had spent literally half my life at the same teaching hospital where I was a professor of psychiatry, a palliative medicine researcher, and the recipient of my Academy's life-time achievement award. Happily married to the same remarkable woman for more than four decades and the father of two children who each made me feel optimistic about the fate of the planet, I was comfortable quietly shutting my office door for the last time. I also had a writing project to pursue—this book—which had quietly begun gestating two years earlier following a dawning appreciation that I was losing my cognitive edge.

Age-related memory lapses or dementia? It remains unclear.

However, I have witnessed others, including family members, who plummeted down the rabbit hole of a dementing illness. And I have concluded that, for me, this would be a fate worse than death. And if this is the case then I have asked myself whether it makes sense to foreshorten one's life upon or after receiving such a diagnosis. And by foreshortening life, I mean get off the bus, accelerate dying, hasten death, kill yourself, commit suicide—basically, pick whatever words with which you are most comfortable.

But few people who fear contracting dementias have given serious thought to whether or how to end life effectively, painlessly, and quickly. Many proclaim, "I'd rather be dead!"—braggadocio comes to mind—but that is hardly the same thing as dispassionately examining the different options, actively preparing, and selecting a time.

Further complicating matters, when it comes to dementia, the default position of healthcare professionals is to order more procedures; to fine-tune the diagnosis; encourage hope; suggest a visit to a spiritual advisor, religious leader, or psychotherapist; tout the value of peer support groups; and/or recommend enrollment in a research study. It is the exceedingly rare doctor, nurse, or other staff person who is willing to invest time conversing about dying—let alone about a wish to kill oneself. Relatively few medical professionals can offer useful information or actively respond to an earnest request for help in truncating life by a rational human being faced with a nightmarish future existence. My colleagues have not usually formulated how they, themselves, might respond to receiving such a diagnosis and, for that matter, who or where they would turn to if they were eager to die.

Upon starting this writing project, my hope has always been that the book might clarify such matters and stimulate conversations between people *and* their families *and* their healthcare providers about these taboo topics. Which is why I still can't get over my incredible luck in having met Dan Winter and his spouse.

Dan wished people might reflect on the words of Dr. Tim Quill that "continued meaningless existence with no escape can become the enemy, and death can be a welcome friend."[1] This was the key to Dan's determination to control Alzheimer's disease by dying, and it is why he eagerly wanted his fellow citizens to learn about the steps that he would take, along with any missteps.

Dan was unafraid to be a trailblazer, and he invited me to accompany him on his journey as an embedded journalist. I marched along with him—curious and sometimes uncomfortable—as he encountered barriers and forks in the road on the way to his destination. Agreeing to join him was the first of three unusual decisions that I made.

The second was to disseminate small sections of the manuscript's narrative to about one hundred palliative care professionals, neurologists, bioethicists, medical aid in dying practitioners, nurses, psychiatrists, geriatricians, science writers, social workers, law professors, social activists, family caregivers, and patients. I was optimistic that specific events would resonate with their professional and personal experiences or, alternatively, strike them as wrong-headed and even offensive. I encouraged them to lend their voices to this project and, like Dan, to be honest and forthright in expressing opinions. However, I never anticipated how enlightening and just plain fun it would be to interview and hear from the multitude of authorities and to learn their reasons for supporting, challenging, or commiserating over this chronicle. Fun—but also frustrating—as they often contradicted each other in a manner that could cause one's head to spin 360 degrees, like the unfortunate young girl in *The Exorcist*.

The third decision has been to construct *Winter's End* for both professional and lay readerships. I did this despite anticipating that the former might complain that scholarly books ought to be more serious, fact-filled, and sober-minded, and the latter would grumble about the distractions posed by the

---

[1] T. Quill, *Death and Dignity: Making Choices and Taking Charge* (New York: Norton, 1993), 25. (First paperback edition, 1994.)

inclusion of information about genetics, pharmacology, and the contradictory opinions of the bioethicists and other authorities. Naturally, my hope remains that both constituencies will find Dan's story sufficiently engrossing that they end up feeling satisfied.

I would like to make it explicit that the purpose of this book has never been to encourage people who dread dementia to kill themselves. I do not intend to lead the reader to any specific conclusion or course of action. Dan, his spouse, and I began the journey knowing that most individuals—whether or not they have a dementia—have an all-powerful survival instinct. We humans adapt to almost everything thrown at us, and we rarely encounter deal-breakers. It is practically unthinkable to genuinely contemplate foreshortening life, especially if one regularly attends religious services where priests, ministers, imams, and rabbis proclaim such actions to be strictly forbidden, selfish, and sinful. Add to this mix one's friends and loving family members, who in most instances will offer arguments in favor of staying the course. *Winter's End* is calculated to bring to the surface the ambiguities, as well as the practical and moral ramifications, of death-hastening decisions.

I hope the book will offer an indelible portrait of its protagonist, a man in possession of remarkable strength and courage, but one who was also subject to human foibles, weaknesses, and failures. I found Dan to be thoughtful, charismatic, and eloquent. However, there was an element of unpredictability that coursed through our interviews, as I realized that, at any moment, Alzheimer's threatened to sweep in like a low-pressure weather system, produce fierce storms, and strip away the sandy beach to reveal bare bedrock beneath.

Throughout this writing project, I have aspired to underscore what the poet Edward Hirsch calls "the foundational importance of free inquiry, original thought, and intellectual autonomy" (email of December 22, 2022). The ideas and sentiments expressed by the many individuals who I quoted are their own and do not reflect the official views of the institutions and professional organizations with which they are affiliated. Naturally, all errors, misquotations, and similar problems are my responsibility solely.

Are there really fates worse than death? Like most people, Dan Winter was uncertain. That is until he visited his father at a memory care unit in Lawrence, Kansas.

Dan's father had been diagnosed with Alzheimer's disease at the age of 70. Winton "Wint" Allen Winter Sr. survived for 13 years, spending his final days, in 2013, at a specialized chronic care facility. Dan remembers sitting silently beside him. His dad, who had once exuberantly embraced life, was unable to speak, understand the simplest words, or make eye contact. He couldn't respond to his name. He was incontinent of bowel and bladder. Wint, like many patients in the final stages of dementia, had even tragically lost the ability to smile.

Dan felt demoralized that his father's formerly agile mind had wound completely down. There was not the slightest whiff of his silly humor, constant state of motion, sometimes irritating logic, or obsession with the Kansas Jayhawks basketball team. Gone were the man's ambitions, yearnings, and capacity to love. To Dan, it seemed that the disease had stripped his dad not only of individuality and personhood, but of his essential humanity.

Wint had been a successful entrepreneur, banker, and cattle rancher. He had faithfully served in the Kansas Senate, where he was known to be articulate, popular, but also sometimes harshly opinionated.

At the nursing facility, Dan looked at the withered man lying in bed and concluded, *There was no him. It was lights out.*

The philosopher, Kwame Anthony Appiah, calls such experiences "a special heartbreak that arises from the doubleness of someone's being here but not here."[1] Appiah would later write: "We are . . . entitled to decide that losing the

---

[1] Appiah KA. The Ethicist: My stepdad has Alzheimer's. Can my mom date someone else? *New York Times.* August 31, 2021, https://www.nytimes.com/2021/08/31/magazine/alzheimers-ethics.html#:~:text=There's%20a%20special%20heartbreak%20that,many%20marriages%20end%20in%20divorce.

cognitive functions necessary for a life of autonomy deprives us of the possibility of a dignified existence. And so we're entitled, in my view, to make plans to end our lives when that happens."[2]

Author Katie Engelhart has recounted the true story of a group of older women who shared Appiah's belief and were sufficiently traumatized by their experiences witnessing family members and friends with dementing illnesses that they created a secret pact. They agreed, "the first one who gets Alzheimer's gets killed by the rest of us."[3,4]

Dan's heart may have been broken, but he was enraged as he gazed at his father. He explained, "Had my dad been able to see himself, he would have been horrified. Had he been able to see his decimated state that day, I'm quite certain he would have been angrier than me."

Dan arrived at the same conclusion as renown filmmaker Luis Buñuel, who exclaimed, "Life without memory is no life at all."[5] Dan made a silent vow: he would never follow his father's example and merely endure. Like Engelhart's women and their suicide cabal, he vividly remembers thinking, *If I am ever diagnosed with Alzheimer's, I will endeavor to determine the manner and timing of my own death.*

Several months later, Wint fell and fractured his hip. It was a bad break, and the family hesitantly agreed with the medical team's recommendation that it be surgically repaired.

Dan arrived at the hospital just as the surgeon reported: "It was a very successful operation. We're really proud of what we did." Turning to Dan and his brother, the physician concluded, "Just make sure he never puts more than 30 percent of his body weight on the leg."

While patently absurd to expect an individual with severe dementia to be capable of following such a dictate, the request turned out to be moot: Wint would never stand upright again. He would die three days later.

After the death, Dan looked around at his family and thought, *We weren't sorry that he died. We were glad he was gone.*

[2] Kwame Anthony Appiah, "The Ethicist: My husband is facing dementia. Can I help him end his life?" *The New York Times*, October 6, 2023. https://www.nytimes.com/2023/10/06/magazine/dementia-suicide-ethics.html

[3] Katie Engelhart, *The Inevitable: Dispatches on the Right to Die* (New York: MacMillan, 2021).

[4] Paige Sutherland, Meghna Chakrabarti, and Tim Skoog, "How the medical aid in dying movement is gaining momentum in the U.S.," *On Point*, May 31, 2023, https://www.wbur.org/onpoint/2023/05/31/how-the-medical-aid-in-dying-movement-is-gaining-momentum-in-the-u-s.

[5] "Quotable quote," Good Reads, accessed June 23, 2023, https://www.goodreads.com/quotes/357380-you-have-to-begin-to-lose-your-memory-if-only.

When Dan recounted this anecdote, he said, "Of course I couldn't say that to just anybody, because people would think I was a callous asshole. But we were relieved this ordeal was over. It was over for him and for us."

Listening to Dan's words, I admired his frankness. *This man doesn't pull any punches*, I thought. And I wondered then, and in every subsequent interview over the succeeding months, *How will it turn out? What lessons will he convey? What can be deciphered from his experiences?*

*****

Arguably among the worst of all medical afflictions, the dementias are a slow-motion tsunami that destroys one's personality; takes a tremendous emotional, physical, and financial toll on patients and families; and are irreversible and inexorably fatal.[6] Alzheimer's disease, the most common type of dementia, begins 20 years or more before memory loss and its other core symptoms become manifest.[7] Approximately 910,000 people aged 65 or older developed Alzheimer's in a single year in the United States.[8] In 2023, there were an estimated 6.7 million Americans aged 65 and older living with Alzheimer's.[9,10] Approximately 200,000 of them, like Dan, carry the diagnosis of younger-onset Alzheimer's disease.[11]

According to the Alzheimer's Association, deaths have more than doubled between 2000 and 2019, while those from heart disease—the leading cause of mortality in the United States—have decreased.[12] The dementias kill more

[6] Karen Harrison Dening, Elizabeth L Sampson, and Kay De Vries, "Advance care planning in dementia: Recommendations for healthcare professionals," *Palliative Care* (February 2019): 12:1178224219826579. doi: 10.1177/1178224219826579. PMID: 30833812; PMCID: PMC6393818.

[7] Clifford R. Jack Jr, Val J. Lowe, Stephen D. Weigand, et al., "Serial PiB and MRI in normal, mild cognitive impairment and Alzheimer's disease: Implications for sequence of pathological events in Alzheimer's disease," *Brain* 132, no. 5 (May 2009): 1355–1365, doi: 10.1093/brain/awp062.

[8] Kumar B. Rajan, Jennifer Weuve, Lisa L. Barnes, Robert S. Wilson, and Denis A Evans, "Prevalence and incidence of clinically diagnosed Alzheimer's disease dementia from 1994 to 2012 in a population study," *Alzheimers & Dementia* 15, no. 1 (January 2019): 1–7, doi: 10.1016/j.jalz.2018.07.216.

[9] "2023 Alzheimer's disease facts and figures," Alzheimer's Association, accessed May 31, 2023, https://www.alz.org/media/documents/alzheimers-facts-and-figures.pdf.

[10] Kumar B. Rajan, Jennifer Weuve, Lisa L. Barnes, Elizabeth A. McAninch, Robert S. Wilson, and Denis A. Evans, "Population estimate of people with clinical AD and mild cognitive impairment in the United States (2020–2060)," *Alzheimers & Dementia* 17, no. 12 (December 2021):1966–1975, doi: 10.1002/alz.12362.

[11] Stevie Hendriks, Kirsten Peetoom, Christian Bakker, et al., "Global prevalence of young-onset dementia: A systematic review and meta-analysis," *JAMA Neurology* 78, no. 9 (September 2021): 1080–1090, doi: 10.1001/jamaneurol.2021.2161.

[12] "Alzheimer's disease facts and figures," Alzheimer's Association, accessed April 17, 2023, https://www.alz.org/alzheimers-dementia/facts-figures?utm_source=google&utm_med

people than breast cancer and prostate cancer combined. They rank sixth among causes of death for white Americans and fourth for Black Americans.[13] During the coronavirus pandemic, the mortality rate dramatically surged.[14]

Yet meaningful data are lacking about how people with dementia develop their constellation of symptoms and how they die.[15-20] The science journalist Robin Marantz Henig has written that when an individual is diagnosed with Alzheimer's disease, "it's hard to know exactly what the trajectory is going to be."[21] Henig also points out, "They really can't predict well whether you're going to be an empty shell or a kinder, gentler, more living-in-the-moment kind of person."

She has highlighted (interview of April 8, 2020) that some individuals with dementias appear to achieve a certain kind of majesty. There are "people who watch their loved ones slip away, or people who go through that slipping-away themselves and are surprised to find a kind of grace in it: the Zen-like existence in an eternal now, the softening of hard edges, the glorification of simple pleasures."

But Dan held an altogether different belief when it came to the memory and cognitive disorders—a view that I share. Our thoughts gravitate to those unfortunate people who become uncontrollably anxious, mix up day and night, develop jealous delusions or become paranoid, wander away from home, and unexpectedly explode with rage. Our stance is that much—although certainly

ium=paidsearch&utm_campaign=google_grants&utm_content=alzheimers&gad=1&gclid=EAIaIQobChMIts_OucCu_gIVwejjBx3OGgx0EAAYASAAEgI1x_D_BwE.

[13] "2022 Alzheimer's disease facts and figures," Alzheimer's Association, accessed September 23, 2022, https://www.alz.org/media/documents/alzheimers-facts-and-figures.pdf.

[14] Lauren Gilstrap, Weiping Zhou, Marcella Alsan, Anoop Nanda, Jonathan S. Skinner, et al., "Trends in mortality rates among Medicare enrollees with Alzheimer disease and related dementias before and during the early phase of the COVID-19 pandemic," *JAMA Neurology* 79, no. 4 (2022):342–348. doi:10.1001/jamaneurol.2022.0010.

[15] S. L. Mitchell, D. K. Kiely, M. B. Hamel, P. S. Park, J. N. Morris, and B. E. Fries, "Estimating prognosis for nursing home residents with advanced dementia," *JAMA*. 291 (2004): 2734–2740.

[16] P. Hanrahan and D. Luchins, "Feasible criteria for enrolling end-stage dementia patients in home hospice care," *The Hospice Journal* 10 (1995): 47–54.

[17] R. S. Schonwetter, B. Han, B. J. Small, B. Martin, K. Tope, and W. E. Haley. "Predictors of six-month survival among patients with dementia: An evaluation of hospice Medicare guidelines," *American Journal of Hospice and Palliative Care* 20 (2003): 105–113.

[18] U. Guehne, S. Riedel-Heller, and M. C. Angermeyer, "Mortality in dementia," *Neuroepidemiology* 25 (2005): 153–162.

[19] H. Brodaty, C. McGilchrist, L. Harris, and K. E. Peters, "Time until institutionalization and death in patients with dementia," *Archives of Neurology* 50 (1993): 643–650.

[20] P. van Dijk, D. Dippel, and J. Habbema, "Survival of patients with dementia," *Journal of the American Geriatric Society* 39 (1991): 603–610.

[21] Robin Marantz Henig, "The last day of her life," *The New York Times*, accessed July 26, 2022, https://www.nytimes.com/2015/05/17/magazine/the-last-day-of-her-life.html.

not all—of the value of human life is determined by a person's mind—the ability to remember and think clearly, the display of a sense of humor, the facility for empathy, along with the continuing capacity to contribute to the welfare of others. He and I would posit that how we die is a crucial element of our legacy, and people should have the right to hasten death. And, last, that the answer to the question, "Am I still me when I have forgotten who I am, and when I no longer remember my dearest ones?" is, unfortunately, "No!"

The above statements are bound to aggravate a lot of people, including a substantial number of ethicists and theologians. Tia Powell, MD, a professor of psychiatry and bioethics at the Albert Einstein College of Medicine in New York told me, "I think you can have a life with dementia that has joy in it, and we need to make sure that's not an empty promise, but an actual one."[22] When we spoke (July 26, 2022), she pointed out, "the stigma against people with dementia is unbelievable." Dr. Powell was clearly concerned whether Dan and I were perpetuating the prejudice of ableism—discrimination "based on the belief that typical abilities are superior, [and] disabled people require 'fixing.'"[23,24]

"Here's my two cents," she exclaimed after reading Dan and my words pertaining to the value of human life—which I now see as possibly sounding glib but not being entirely wrong. "Tying human worth (or personhood) to cognitive capacity has been questioned and strongly rejected by many."[25]

Dr. Powell went on to say, "The strongest argument in favor of aid in dying for those with dementia is likely to rely on their real-time suffering—and certainly not that they are less human and less valued than they once were."

In that same vein, Dr. Marzena Gieniusz, medical director of the Alzheimer's and Dementia Care Program at Northwell Health adds, "It's important to help patients and their loved ones understand that it's not hopeless, and there are always things we can do to help manage the disease, despite being unable to stop its progression or reverse the disease process."[26]

[22] Edie Grossfield, "Dementia care reimagined: A Q&A with Dr. Tia Powell," NextAvenue, accessed July 28, 2022, https://www.nextavenue.org/dementia-care-reimagined-tia-powell/.

[23] Ashley Eisenmenger, "Ableism 101: What it is, what it looks like, and what we can do to to fix it," Access Living, accessed July 30, 2020, https://www.accessliving.org/newsroom/blog/ableism-101/.

[24] Joseph Vukov, "Personhood and natural kinds: Why cognitive status need not affect moral status," *Journal of Medical Philosophy* 42, no. 3 (June 2017): 261–277, doi:10.1093/jmp/jhx005.

[25] Stephen G. Post, "Respectare: Moral respect for the lives of the deeply forgetful," in Julian Hughes, Stephen Louw, and Steven R Sabat (eds.), *Dementia: Mind, Meaning, and the Person, International Perspectives in Philosophy & Psychiatry* (Oxford University Press, 2005), 223–234, https://doi.org/10.1093/med/9780198566151.003.0014.

[26] Steven Reinberg, "Suicide risk rises sharply in people diagnosed with early-onset dementia," U.S. News & World Report, accessed October 6, 2022, https://www.usnews.com/news/health-news/articles/2022-10-04/suicide-risk-rises-sharply-in-people-diagnosed-with-early-onset-dementia.

According to Father Tadeusz Pacholczyk, PhD: "As the symptoms and complications of dementia unfold, the challenges we face from the disease can unexpectedly become an invitation from God. . . . Such moments, nevertheless, offer important opportunities to grow in grace, to slow down, to reevaluate our priorities, and to enter into a more profound relationship with Him who is our final destination and abiding hope."[27]

From a secular perspective, Jeremy Hughes, chief executive of the United Kingdom's Alzheimer's Society, has written: "We want to reassure people that life doesn't end when dementia begins. We know that dementia is the most feared health condition of our time and there's no question that it can have a profound and devastating impact on people, their family and friends—but getting a timely diagnosis will enable people with dementia to live as well as possible."[28]

As well as possible?

While I mostly agree with the thrust of the above statements, at the same time, I'm not ready to wag my finger and dispute it when someone like Dan tells me that their disease has left him feeling lessened in our hypercognitive world. Or that he would always be horrified at how it ravaged his father and destroyed the essence of the man he had known. Dan's viewpoint resonates with the message of Rebecca Solnit's memoir, where she writes: "The self is also a creation, the principal work of your life, the crafting of which makes everyone an artist."[29]

Dan was an art lover, and he unfortunately witnessed how dementia erased his father's bold, artistic creation of a self. Wint had been the family patriarch, a political leader, and an inspiring giant of a man. The disease reduced him to a shell. He may not have loudly railed or become psychotic, but for years he became a husk of his former self. Dan's position is that our culture highly values individual freedom, and, unless this violates the rights of others, persons should be free to choose how they want to live their lives, including the terminus of those lives.[30,31]

*****

[27] Tadeusz Pacholoczyk, "Seeking the spiritual side of dementia," Echoes, accessed November 6, 2022, https://thebostonpilot.com/Opinion/article.asp?ID=193542.

[28] "Over half of people fear dementia diagnosis, 62 per cent think it means 'life is over,'" Alzheimer's Society, accessed October 8, 2020, https://www.alzheimers.org.uk/news/2018-05-29/over-half-people-fear-dementia-diagnosis-62-cent-think-it-means-life-over.

[29] Rebecca Solnit, *The Faraway Nearby* (New York: Viking Books, 2013).

[30] Douglas W. Heinrichs, "The case for medical assistance in dying: Part 1," *Psychiatric Times*, accessed August 31, 2022, https://www.psychiatrictimes.com/view/the-case-for-medical-aid-in-dying-part-1.

[31] Sebastian Junger, *Freedom* (New York: Simon & Schuster, 2021).

Some hard facts to hear?

Alzheimer's disease and the other dementias don't just make people forgetful. They are serious, progressive conditions which are eventually fatal. In the United Kingdom, the United States, and other privileged countries, it is estimated that one in three people over the age of 65 will die with or from one of the dementias.[32-34] According to the Australian Associated Press, the neurodegenerative disorders have overtaken coronary heart disease as the leading cause of illness, injury, and death among Australians aged 65 and over.[35] Dementia accounts for almost 10% of deaths in Australia, and it's the thing that women aged 75 or more are most likely die from.[36]

In the United Kingdom, Wendy Mitchell, a former National Health Service administrator with young-onset vascular dementia and Alzheimer's disease for the past nine years, cautions that an aid-in-dying bill has not passed despite repeated efforts. She points out that, under the terms of the Suicide Act (1961), assisted suicide continues to be punishable by up to 14 years' imprisonment.[37] Mitchell writes that "choice . . . is at the centre of everything we do as humans every day—or at least those of us lucky enough to enjoy the choice of bodily autonomy and who are not bound by regimes or other strict diktats." Echoing Dan, she concludes, "And yet, we have no choice over when we die, or at least we don't in the country I live in."

When Dying With Dignity Victoria surveyed the views of its members on their country's current assisted dying law, the comments were filled with pleas for

[32] Carol Brayne, Lu Gao, Michael Dewey, Fiona E. Matthews, and Medical Research Council Cognitive Function and Ageing Study Investigators, "Dementia before death in ageing societies: The promise of prevention and the reality," *PLoS Med* 3, no. 10 (October 2006): e397. PMID: 17076551 PMCID: PMC1626550 DOI: 10.1371/journal.pmed.0030397.

[33] Ralph Jones, "Book review: O, Let Me Not Get Alzheimer's, Sweet Heaven!: Dementia is the most common cause of death in England and Wales. Should sufferers have the right to end their own lives?," New Humanist, accessed October 14, 2022, https://newhumanist.org.uk/articles/5702/book-review-o-let-me-not-get-alzheimers-sweet-heaven.

[34] "Statistical bulletin: Deaths registered in England and Wales; (series DR)," Office for National Statistics (ONS), 2017, accessed January 3, 2019, https://www.ons.gov.uk/peoplepopulationandcommunity/birthsdeathsandmarriages/deaths/bulletins/deathsregisteredinenglandandwalesseriesdr/2016#dementia-and-alzheimer-disease-remained-the-leading-cause-of-death-in-2016.

[35] Mibenge Nsenduluka, "Dementia now afflicts more seniors than heart disease," *Illawarra Mercury*, February 22, 2023, https://www.illawarramercury.com.au/story/8096642/dementia-now-afflicts-more-seniors-than-heart-disease/.

[36] "Euthanasia law review must consider the thorny issue of dementia," *The Age*, accessed June 14, 2023, https://www.theage.com.au/politics/victoria/euthanasia-law-review-must-consider-the-thorny-issue-of-dementia-20230613-p5dg45.html.

[37] Kat Lister, "'We need to talk about the end': Wendy Mitchell on living positively with Alzheimer's," *The Guardian*, accessed June 19, 2023, https://www.theguardian.com/society/2023/jun/18/wendy-mitchell-author-on-living-with-alzheimers.

the statute to be broadened and dementia to be included. This issue in the end-of-life debate is contentious but rapidly gaining support, and the organization's president, Jane Morris has stated, "What we really want to emphasize is that access for dementia sufferers is at the front of mind for Australians."[38] In the article "Slow Torture," journalist Michael Bachelard points out that "in Australia there is no provision for people living with dementia to choose their time of death."[39] Bachelard writes, "This is the monster in the room."[40]

Robin Marantz Henig is correct that, even if we can't cure Alzheimer's disease, it certainly would be helpful if medical research could at least give us a clearer idea of the trajectory of a person's dementia. Patients should have a better idea about the timing of the disease's different stages, what symptoms to expect from their brain damage, and how long they are likely to survive.[41] Furthermore, it would be exceedingly useful to know and track the avenues by which people can die—whether as a result of accidents, treatment withdrawal or withholding, co-existing medical conditions that are neglected, aspiration pneumonia, inanition, and suicide.[42,43] People who have dementing illnesses, along with their loved ones, ought to be provided with information to allow them to better anticipate the future and make provisions.

I began a series of formal interviews with Dan exactly 9 months before his demise. During this period and the succeeding two years, I also interviewed his husband, John David Forsgren. While Francois de La Rochefoucauld (1678) cautioned that, "Neither the sun nor death can be looked at with a steady eye," both Dan and John demonstrated to me that they are among the

---

[38] Melissa Cunningham, "'People dying during the process': The push to free up Victoria's euthanasia laws," *The Sydney Morning Herald*, accessed June 18, 2023, https://www.smh.com.au/national/victoria/people-dying-during-the-process-the-push-to-free-up-victoria-s-euthanasia-laws-20230614-p5dghz.html.

[39] Michael Bachelard, "'Slow torture': Readers tell how dementia experience shaped their views on voluntary assisted dying," *The Age*, accessed June 12, 2023, https://www.theage.com.au/national/victoria/slow-torture-readers-tell-how-dementia-experience-shaped-their-views-on-voluntary-assisted-dying-20230605-p5de16.html.

[40] Michael Bachelard, "My mother-in-law chose to die with dignity: Dementia sufferers deserve the same right," *The Age*, May 8, 2023, https://www.theage.com.au/national/victoria/my-mother-in-law-chose-to-die-with-dignity-dementia-sufferers-deserve-the-same-right-20230426-p5d3ig.html.

[41] H. Aguero-Torres, L. Fratiglioni, and B. Winblad, "Natural history of Alzheimer's disease and other dementias: Review of the literature in the light of the findings from the Kungsholmen project," *International Journal of Geriatric Psychiatry* 13 (1998): 755–766.

[42] Jane Gilbert, "How does a person die from dementia?," Hometouch, May 5, 2019, https://myhometouch.com/articles/how-does-a-person-die-from-dementia.

[43] Jane Gilbert, "How does a person die from dementia?," Hometouch, May 5, 2019, https://myhometouch.com/articles/how-does-a-person-die-from-dementia.

remarkable human beings who share the capacity to contemplate their own nonexistence.[44,45]

From the first, it was apparent that Dan resolutely wished to abbreviate his suffering from Alzheimer's disease, and he was sorely disappointed at being ineligible to receive legal, medical aid-in-dying. He decided if this method wasn't available in the United States, then he wanted to find another escape hatch. *Winter's End* is intended to be a scholarly account of Dan's quest to achieve what he considered to be a good and authentic death. I was never planning on writing a love story, but this book also reveals the two men's touching relationship.

Dan and John made a generous decision to candidly recount the details of their lives to me. This book exposes their fears, desires, heartaches, and frustrations while detailing the agony of the Alzheimer's diagnosis and the ensuing family conflicts, as well as the circumstances underlying Dan's choices.

My intention has been to treat the experience as a scholarly project—a detailed case report—and to learn as much as possible from it. As I came to appreciate how the dementing illnesses are increasingly occurring throughout the world, the book also came to include brief anecdotes based not only in the United States, but also Canada, Asia, and Europe. Many people with dementia do not want to be left behind by the global right-to-die movement; however, there are a host of profound issues that need to be confronted to permit this to rationally occur.

In one sense, *Winter's End* is an enormous thought experiment that asks: If I'm going to be diagnosed with a dementia, can I achieve some degree of control over my life and the terminus of that life? What can I do in advance to prepare? If one is going to set a time "to exit the train," then how can this be determined? What symptoms are intolerable? What are the available "natural" exits? What other methods to hasten death are feasible?

Dan would teach me that many people want to have more end-of-life options and to have the freedom to arrive at their own autonomous decisions. While he had no wish to follow Wint's path, he accepted that what happened to his father is presently more "normative" than what he had in mind for himself. Dan hoped that by expressing his wishes and describing his ensuing journey, he would stimulate readers—be they professionals or lay persons—to openly talk about an otherwise forbidden subject.

[44] "Francois de La Rochefoucauld quotes," Brainy Quotes, accessed June 14, 2023, https://www.brainyquote.com/quotes/francois_de_la_rochefouca_151021.

[45] Maurice Manning, "'Death, like sun cannot be looked at steadily': (François de la Rochefoucauld–1678)," *Studies: An Irish Quarterly Review* 98, no. 392 (Winter 2009): 379–391, https://www.jstor.org/stable/25660701.

   In 1966, when Dr. Elizabeth Kubler Ross first sat down at the bedside of a
dying patient at the University of Chicago, the widely held assumptions were
that terminally ill people didn't want to talk about their imminent deaths and
that such conversations would obliterate hope.[46] These proved to be false.
Having devoted five years to this project, I am confident that there are a substantial number of individuals, like Dan and John, who are eager to engage in conversation about the different means to shorten or to maintain life in the context
of dementia. There are plenty of people who don't wish to passively relinquish
control over the end.

---

[46] Elisabeth Kübler-Ross, *On Death and Dying: What the Dying Have to Teach Doctors, Nurses,
Clergy, and Their Own Families* (New York: Scribner; Reissue edition, 2014).

2

I first encountered Dan while watching a webinar in April of 2020.[1] The organization, Compassion & Choices (C&C), which co-produced the event, had launched an initiative to encourage people with dementias to think about their final phase of life, the choices they could potentially make, and the benefits of discussing them with loved ones. The nonprofit had developed a "Dementia Values & Priorities Tool."[2] This online instrument described the stages of dementia, and it then explored an individual's personal values, quality of life concerns, and whether he or she wanted every available medical treatment—no matter the circumstances. Alternatively, it inquired about whether there was a point after which they would want to be kept comfortable and be "allowed to die naturally."

Dan was part of a four-person panel. In the webinar, he praised C&C's tool and explained: "I feel I have some much-needed control around my death . . . before I lose my capacity to make decisions for myself. I can now face the practical questions that surround the rest of my life. For instance, I let my driver's license expire in August because I didn't want family members to have to force me to do so as my disease advances and when I may not be thinking straight about the risks that I present to others behind the wheel. That's just one small example of the type of considerations the Toolkit provided me. It encouraged me. It made me think. And the ability to think about the plan for my death is a great comfort to me."

[1] "Living and dying with dementia: Taking charge of your personal values," Compassion & Choices, accessed July 28, 2022, https://compassionandchoices.org/take-action/staying-stronger-together/living-and-dying-with-dementia-webinar/.

[2] "Dementia values and priorities tool," Compassion & Choices, accessed July 28, 2022, https://values-tool.compassionandchoices.org/?_ga=2.115898886.1491350545.1649859175-964474418.1649173599.

With considerable dignity, he told the 500 participants who tuned in, "Now I can be upfront about the intentional life I want to lead from here on. I'm also upfront about the death I want and the death I don't want. I want to outsmart my disease and deny it the ability to erase my own personhood during the last lap."

He concluded his presentation by saying, "I now have choices that I didn't know that I had—like the ability to live until the last day of my life with a sense of grace and choice. Because for me, on my last day, I want to feel the love. Thank you."

Dan's message stirred me deeply, and I decided to seek him out to learn more.

It proved to be a relatively simple matter to track down his contact information and arrange for our first formal interview. From the start, he encouraged me to also speak with his husband, John, and made it clear they were life partners. Within the first few minutes of my conversations with the two men—each of whom I repeatedly spoke with separately—I understood that Dan intended to quicken his death.

Dan agreed to give me a very rare, if not unprecedented, access to his story as it was happening and to provide me with introductions to others in his life. Dan's journey would come to involve many fascinating and sometimes unexpected twists and turns, and he hoped that together we would paint a multifaceted portrait depicting how patients with dementia might wish to die.

*****

"How do we do this?" Dan asked from his home in Portland, Oregon.

"You talk, and I'll listen," I answered, having telephoned him from my cabin on a lake in Western Massachusetts.

"Okay, then I'll tell you about my bathroom," he replied.

This statement left me worried about what I might have gotten myself into.

I knew that he had been diagnosed with a dementia some 3 years earlier and was actively trying to circumnavigate the disease. But I now became concerned whether in the good-humored but spooky words of author Stephen King, he was "riding into the Kingdom of Dementia on the Alzheimer's Express."[3]

[3] Stephen King, *Mr. Mercedes: A Novel* (New York: Pocket Books, 2015), 88, Google Books, https://books.google.com/books?id=_l5BCwAAQBAJ&pg=PA88&lpg=PA88&dq=mr.+merce des+riding+into+the+kingdom+of+dementia+on+the+alzheimer%27s+express&source= bl&ots=0mV4srszdq&sig=ACfU3U1W3fona8zOprOhEO6bk4phvrENDA&hl=en&sa=X&ved= 2ahUKEwicgOD056P5AhVcrIkEHV7qAOYQ6AF6BAgCEAM#v=onepage&q=mr.%20merce des%20riding%20into%20the%20kingdom%20of%20dementia%20on%20the%20alzheimer's%20 express&f = false.

However, it turned out Dan wanted to tell me about the "memory mirror" he had constructed on a bathroom wall, which was covered with snapshots and memorabilia.

"Are you in a position to walk into the bathroom right now and describe it to me?" I asked. It was 2020. For this and all subsequent interviews, I resisted using videoconferencing, as I preferred keeping the focus on his words, ideas, and emotions.

"Yup," Dan replied, "and I'll attach a couple of pictures to an email later. I may make it sound like Valhalla," he chuckled, "but it's a bathroom and also functions as our laundry room.

"Here are some street photographs of me with each of my three kids at roughly the same age. There's a photograph of all the women who are closest to me—my two sisters, my two sisters-in-law, and my ex-wife."

He took a breath. "I've got a photograph of two of my dogs. I've got a separate photograph of my dad, his sister, and me. There's one of my favorites—a recent photograph of my mother, at age 86, accepting an award from the hospital in our town for her many years of service and. . . . "

"Service in what capacity?" I interrupted.

Dan responded, "She was the president of a hospital auxiliary that raised money for a new wing, and she also gave money to put in a chapel." Dan added that he came from a traditional, Catholic family.

"Over here," he said, "is a photograph of my two grandmothers. Neither of them liked me." From our earliest interactions, it was apparent that directness is one of Dan's defining attributes.

"There's a picture of my two youngest children at the beach. Is that the cutest fucking thing you've ever seen in your life?" he asked, forgetting for a moment I couldn't see the photo. I learned that it was rare for him to swear during our interviews, and I couldn't help but wonder whether his executive function—specifically his self-control—was slipping.

"Let's see," Dan continued. "Here is a Maya Angelou quote from one of her poems: 'When we come to it. When we let the rifles fall from our shoulders.' Do you know this passage?"

"No, I don't."

"Okay if I recite it to you?"

"Sure."

"One stanza goes: '*When we come to It / When we let the rifles fall from our shoulders / And children dress their dolls in flags of truce / When land mines of death have been removed / And the aged can walk into evenings of peace / When religious ritual is not perfumed / By the incense of burning flesh / And childhood dreams are not kicked awake / By nightmares of abuse.*'"

"What does that Maya Angelou piece mean to you?" I asked. "Why do you have that up on the mirror?"

"I'm a survivor of child abuse," he explained. I could feel the emotional tone of the interview darken. He went on to say, "She references that at the end of this passage." And then Dan distinctly lightened the mood with the comment, "But it's such a lovely, mellifluous way of describing horrific things. It's horrible and uplifting and beautiful. It's a genius piece of writing."

Shifting back to the mirror, he said: "This is the photograph of a second home our family has in Taos, New Mexico. Now, there's a little snapshot that shows the door of a pickup truck, which says, 'OK Ranch, Junction City.' It is a 15,000-acre working cattle ranch in central western Kansas that was a big part of my upbringing."

I pondered what it must be like to have a family ranch—the Winter's actually had three ranches that extended into different states—and for an adolescent to spend his summers working alongside cowboys. Dan's children, who mainly knew their father as a banker dressed in conservative suits, have likewise had a difficult time conceiving of him laboring at the OK Ranch. However, those were among Dan's happiest times, immersed in a Kansas locale described as being "more the West than Middle West."[4] It was a place where the local accent was "barbed with a prairie twang, a ranch-hand nasalness, and the men, many of them, wear narrow frontier trousers, Stetsons, and high-heeled boots with pointed toes."

Dan paused to reflect on his memories. Once again alluding to the mirror's adornments, he said with considerable warmth, "Of course, there are several pictures of John."

I couldn't see his face but imagined him smiling, as he summed up, "Good times! Yup, good times!"

These are autobiographical Post-It Notes, I thought. *Even if I don't yet know how they are connected, Dan is displaying and telling me about his life's high points.*

He continued, "I work these photographs into my day, every day, whether I kind of know it or not."

"What do you mean you work them into your day?"

"I look at them. I appreciate them. I enjoy them. It's a little narcissistic because I'm in most of these. But I'm also in them with. . . . There's nobody pictured here dead or alive that I wouldn't want to be with."

---

[4] Truman Capote, *In Cold Blood: A True Account of a Multiple Murder and Its Consequences* (New York: Random House, 1966), 1.

"Nice," I said. Unsuccessfully, I tried to explain to him how this moved me. How it seemed like he was constructing art, fabricating, and stringing together pieces of life. I really liked that he was *working it* into his day.

Dan remarked: "I've never been one to traffic in sayings or canards. But I have got something on the mirror that says, 'I promise to live a life so rich of love that at the end, I would not be so shy of death.'"

Dan raced along, mentioning a felt patch from his high school leather jacket that proudly proclaimed, "The Ottawa Kansas Cyclones are the 1973 Eastern Kansas League Champions"; a diminutive copy of a favorite painting by Albert Looking Elk from Taos, New Mexico; his appreciation of the singer Whitney Houston; a snapshot of the ballet dancer Jacques d'Amboise; and so on.

But I was stuck and couldn't disengage myself from the quote promising *to live a life so rich in love that at the end, I would not be so shy of death.* Google reveals it's by the Canadian Instagram poet known as Atticus, who also wrote: "Break my heart and you will find yourself inside."

As for me, Dan was breaking my heart, and I could feel my eyes brimming over with tears.

Like many people, I have a refrigerator at home decorated with photographs and magnets. Until now, I hadn't given it much thought or considered that it might also be a private shrine. But having heard Dan's musings, I began thinking about time, humor, continuity, and the centrality of family. Plus, how the displays on our fridges are archeological fragments—broken pottery shards that, reassembled and pasted back together, may turn out to be an ancient Greek vase.

Fifteen minutes earlier, when I had first rung Dan's cell phone, he was confused about which button to push. But the man could still be thoughtful and eloquent. That is Alzheimer's disease in its early stage. Dan, 61, and his husband, John, 69, were weathering the 2020 election turmoil, partisan divisions, and noisy protests that battered the center of Portland, just a few blocks from their apartment. Despite the social unrest, dementia was justifiably centermost on the minds of the two men.

"Everybody thinks this disease is about memory," Dan said. "It is about memory, but it's also about context. I simply don't get the context of some things that are pretty simple. So, I might give an inappropriate or unrelated response to a question or a comment. If the question is about donuts, I'll give you an answer about windows. . . . And that concept writ large takes up an awful lot of my day. Trying to figure out, *What did I just hear?* or *What did I just read?* I know I need to respond, but I can't find the right context."

3

When I asked Joseph J. Fins, MD, the Chief of the Division of Medical Ethics at Weill Cornell Medical College and current President of the International Neuroethics Society, to review the previous chapter, what jumped off the page for him was the word "context."

He was greatly moved (interview on July 28, 2022) at the thought of Dan "losing his context," and Dr. Fins told me, "It's the photographs, it's the pictures, it's the embeddedness of this person in a life that's slipping away. We're crafted as individuals in the context of our families. It is our families that make us, and we make our families. Dan's context is dissolving, and those relationships are still there sentimentally, but they are slipping away." Dr. Fins evoked the image of how when the ink runs low on our printer cartridges the succeeding pages get fainter, and "then you barely can see the print. And that's how these relationships kind of vanish until they're no longer there."

I thought to myself that Alzheimer's disease is a strange illness, reaching in like a pair of invisible scissors, repeatedly and slowly over time severing connections between the important and unimportant things in our lives and, most heartrendingly, the key people in our lives. I had not previously considered the tragedy of a slowly collapsing context.

Half of Americans aged 40 and older suspect they will be diagnosed with Alzheimer's.[1] A few of them hope that they will be able to actively prepare to cut short their lives and prevent unbearable suffering. To accomplish this, though, a plan needs to be in place before the disease gathers enough momentum to make such a course of action impractical. That is why preparation should ideally take place before diagnosis, by which I mean completing advance (dementia) directives, appointing a healthcare proxy, having discussions with that specific

---

[1] AARP, "Perceptions about dementia don't match reality," accessed July 28, 2022, https://www.aarp.org/research/topics/health/info-2021/dementia-diagnosis-stigma.html.

individual, investigating different death-accelerating methods, and testing the waters with others who may potentially weigh in at the end.

The practical problem is that, before the symptoms crank up and the diagnosis is established, suicide and the ending of life is an intellectual proposition, more theoretical than real. People understandably wish to avoid the catastrophic dementia symptoms, but they aren't ready to *seriously* contemplate ending life and stepping away from family, friends, and the stimulation of work until they absolutely must. They hope the family doctor, a neurologist, or palliative care practitioner will assuage the disease's symptoms, but, realistically, medical professionals can't offer anything substantial to improve one's memory, one's ability to follow conversations, or many of the other dementia phenomena. So, while some unusual individuals may take steps early, much of the preparation will likely occur after diagnosis and during the early stage of the disease.

When we first met, Dan seemed to me to be well positioned to formulate a plan and carry out the resolution he had made while sitting alongside his father at the memory impairment facility—if he didn't wait too long. But just how long was "too long" remained to be seen.

Dan's words were inspiring to me but also frightening. Like many other septuagenarians, I have found that many things no longer automatically fall into place. I recognize the need to rely more on Google to aid my memory or to find workarounds for remembering people's names (such as by surreptitiously elbowing my wife). Verbal recall of conversations that used to be effortless now suddenly tend to freeze up. I no longer remember musical pieces or books that I read years ago. Many gray-haired people hope these things are minor sequelae of aging. But they also anxiously obsess over whether such phenomena might be signs of the memory impairment or damaged executive function of incipient dementia.

The latter is a set of skills essential for planning, organizing information, following directions, and multitasking.[2] If executive function is impaired, then it will impact several different domains of cognition.

In discussing Dan's prognosis and decision to terminate his life, Dr. Fins reminded me that he opposes death-hastening practices—at least when ending life is the primary motivation of the individual or clinician.[3] The relief of suffering and prolongation of life are not always both possible; healing and helping to bring about the terminus of life are mainly contradictory goals.[4] Physicians

---

[2] Knvul Sheikh, "What is brain fog and how can I treat it?," *The New York Times*, September 13, 2022, https://www.nytimes.com/2022/09/13/well/mind/brain-fog-treatment.html.

[3] Joseph J. Fins, *A Palliative Ethic of Care: Clinical Wisdom at Life's End* (Sudbury, MA: Jones and Bartlett, 2006).

[4] Charles McKhann, *A Time to Die: The Place of Physician Assistance* (New Haven, CT: Yale University Press, 1999), 9.

face an irreconcilable ethical dilemma, according to Dr. Fins, who cautioned me that aiding someone to end their life is "not a private or individual act. It's an active one that affects many others and should be understood in the context of family and connectivity. Often, it's cast as this libertarian urge, you know, to control the manner and timing of one's own death. But it's a death in the family. It's a death in a context."

Dr. Fins is hardly alone in believing that the current preeminence accorded to autonomy is a fad and little more than an overblown cultural myth which is frequently imposed on the most vulnerable.[5,6]

Dame Cicely Saunders, a founder of the modern hospice and palliative care movement, famously said, "You matter because you are you, and you matter to the last moment of your life. We will do all we can to not only help you die peacefully, but also to live until you die."[7] Dame Saunders said nothing about any need to be independent, cognitively intact, or productive until the end.

The Lutheran theologian and bioethicists Gilbert Mailanaender is often quoted for his essay, "I want to burden my loved ones."[8] Mailanaender wrote about the many times he chafed under the burdens of teaching his children to play boring games, the endless hours spent at clunky juvenile sporting events and unharmonious piano recitals, the ghastly experiences of being trapped at interminable school plays, his late-night fretting at the bedside of sick kids and of being forced to argue the merits of Burger King versus McDonald's—followed by the Mailanaender family insistence that they then decamp to the fast-food restaurant the young ones had chosen. All of which prompts him to ask: "Why should I *not* be a bit of a burden to these children in my dying?"

His opinion piece has set many people to nodding their heads in agreement.

But there are others who question whether consideration of the burdens dementia imposes on loved ones should be blithely dismissed. Charlotte Raven, an English writer, was diagnosed in 2006 with Huntington disease, just 18 months after the birth of a child. This is a genetic and incurable neurodegenerative disorder that usually becomes evident between the ages of 30 and 50; besides for forgetfulness and impaired judgment, there are often personality changes, severe

   [5] Joshua Briscoe, "Dying, but not alone: We can't escape the social dimension of choosing how we die," The New Atlantis, accessed September 29, 2022, https://www.thenewatlantis.com/publications/dying-but-not-alone.

   [6] David Ames and John Obeid, "Voluntary assisted dying should not be available to dementia patients," The Sydney Morning Herald, June 10, 2023, https://www.smh.com.au/national/voluntary-assisted-dying-should-not-be-available-to-dementia-patients-20230607-p5deqo.html.

   [7] "Cicely Saunders quotes," AZ Quotes, accessed April 25, 2023, https://www.azquotes.com/author/20332-Cicely_Saunders.

   [8] Gilbert Meilaender, "I want to burden my loved ones," First Things, accessed June 10, 2023, https://www.firstthings.com/article/2010/03/i-want-to-burden-my-loved-ones.

mood swings, and chorea (involuntary muscle movements).[9] Raven seriously considered suicide, and she poignantly wrote: "I feared becoming an obstruction to be navigated round: a succubus draining life from the family host. I couldn't stand the thought of my daughter being scared of me. I pictured her dawdling at the top of the street on her way home from school, putting off the moment she would have to confront an irascible and unpredictable parent. I feared I might set fire to the house with her in it, like Woody Guthrie's Huntington disease-affected mother. Or parade in front of her schoolfriends in my underwear."[10]

In Raven's most recent piece, she explains, "I understand now through the visceral experience of my illness that assisted death is not an easy option but a pragmatic solution."[11] She declares that it feels to her like the *best* solution.

I believe Dan's memory mirror attests to the high regard he holds the Winters and that he is not unmindful of the likely impact of a suicide on them. But based on the experience with his father, my impression is that he feels he would be doing both himself and the Winter clan a disservice if he allowed the Alzheimer's disease to relentlessly progress. Dan understands that the lives of our cherished loved ones can be seriously compromised by the very real burdens required to care for people who are increasingly distant, unresponsive, and incapacitated—let alone Raven's concerns about delusions, volatility, and irrational violent outbursts. Whether the cost of caring for patients who have dementing illnesses is emotional, financial, or social—it is usually a combination of all of these—and whether it requires family members to defer or abandon their own desires and needs, it can be overwhelming.

The philosopher John Hardwig has written, "If I end my life to spare the futures of my loved ones, I testify in my death that I am connected to them."[12,13] In the same essay, he also declares, "I believe I may well have a duty to end my life when I can see mental incapacity on the horizon."

[9] "What is Huntington's disease?," Huntington Society of America, accessed April 13, 2023, https://hdsa.org/what-is-hd/overview-of-huntingtons-disease/.

[10] Charlotte Raven, "Charlotte Raven: Should I take my own life?," *The Guardian*, modified April 17, 2010, https://www.theguardian.com/society/2010/jan/16/charlotte-raven-should-i-take-my-own-life.

[11] Charlotte Raven, "Author Charlotte Raven: 'At this point of no return, assisted dying feels like the best solution,'" *The Guardian*, accessed April 10, 2023, https://www.theguardian.com/society/2023/apr/02/author-charlotte-raven-at-this-point-of-no-return-assisted-dying-feels-like-the-best-solution.

[12] "John Hardwig," Wikipedia, accessed August 20, 2022, https://en.wikipedia.org/wiki/John_Hardwig.

[13] John Hardwig, "Some individuals have a duty to die," in *Assisted Suicide*, ed. Laura Egendorf (San Diego: Greenhaven Press Inc., 1998), 199–208.

In short, I respect the opinion of Dr. Fins and his allies that people should be given the opportunity to adapt to dementia and to allow their families the privilege of caring for them—and for many people it *is* a privilege. There are 11.5 million unpaid family caregivers who strive to maintain a positive attitude,[14] like actor Bruce Willis's wife, Emma Hemmings Willis, who recently said, "I have times when I'm in it to win it and times when I can't focus due to life. I try to start my day and end my day in gratitude."[15]

However, Dan's determination to die before Alzheimer's robs him of his identity, his accustomed role within the extended family, and the memories that he has now selected to display on his bathroom wall should not be reflexively dismissed. His wish to die is bound to make us feel uncomfortable, but we can also admire the courage required to fulfil it.

[14] "10 ways Alzheimer's affects family caregivers," *My Prime Time News*, accessed May 30, 2023, https://www.myprimetimenews.com/10-ways-alzheimers-affects-family-caregivers/.

[15] "Bruce Willis' wife claims people are worried and anxious about visiting dementia-stricken star," Ace Showbiz, accessed May 30, 2023, https://www.aceshowbiz.com/news/view/00206 040.html.

4

Dan was a fifth-generation Kansan from a privileged background who, like his father, Wint, led an unusual life.

"Would you send me a few photographs, so I can see what you look like?" I asked at our first meeting—or more accurately, our first pandemic telephone interview.

He laughed and quickly agreed. The resultant attachments reveals him to be a tall, handsome man with steely gray hair parted neatly on the side, glasses with thick dark frames, and an athletic build maintained through daily cycling. But what astounded me the most is his obvious gentleness, mysteriously conveyed in each image, along with a comforting smile.

When I spoke to his friend and neighbor, Pauline Lewis, she could hardly stop gushing over her first encounter with Dan: how imposing he appeared ("You come up to his navel"), his physicality ("The way he moves and everything"), and his charisma ("When you look him in the eye, you can't look away because he's so charming"). But what was most striking to Pauline—and this was all said in the presence of her husband, Drew, who fully agreed—was how Dan immediately attracted people into his circle. He was not only remarkably warm, but, when he spoke with you, he made it clear that no one else was more important.

Pauline said, "For me, it was love at first sight." Quickly glancing at Drew, she clarified, "You know, from a friendship perspective."

Dan's husband, John David Forsgren, slender and quick to smile, answered my question about Dan's appearance by saying: "What does Dan look like? Well, Dan is curly haired and of German extraction. One look and you suspect that's his heritage. . . . He's a really white guy."

Dan is also 6′ 4″, which means that he qualifies for Tall Clubs International, and that means he's frequently asked by strangers whether he used to play basketball.[1] Another member of that organization has a regular tongue-in-cheek response to such enquiries.

"No," he'd say, "did you play miniature golf?"

"It's funny," John continued, "but it took me a long time to realize Dan is much larger than me. I'm 5' 7" on a good day, but I've never thought of myself as being small. And it wasn't until I was with him for a while that I realized he's a lot bigger. He's 240 pounds, and I'm 175 pounds. Because I never felt small, I never felt him to be big. I've never felt overpowered or intimidated by his size. So, in that way, there's grace."

Echoing Pauline, he added: "Dan's one of those people who, when he's talking to you, you are the center of the world. He really listens. And the tragedy of this disease is that he has an extraordinary memory for details about people and their likes and their wants and their experiences. He is also keenly observant about art and fascinated where a piece of art sits in the history of a movement and how it has been influenced by other artists. Very contextual. It boggles one's mind."

Listening to John, I thought, *It is not coincidental that a copy of a beloved painting by Albert Looking Elk is on the magic mirror.*

I also realized, *There's that word, context, again.*

John highlighted how Dan appeared to him in a video from 15 years earlier while addressing a gathering of the American Civil Liberties Union of Kansas. "Man, oh, man, oh, man, he was just firing on all 24 cylinders. His command of information and his ability to give a speech . . . it was really beautiful."

The film, which I later watched, amply demonstrated Dan's qualities as a persuasive, natural leader, and a confident trailblazer.

This is understandable because he is a descendant of trailblazers. "My ancestors," Dan explained, "were farmers and ranchers who originally moved from West Virginia to the Kansas Territory in the 1850s. They homesteaded and helped found the territorial capital of Lecompton. We were some of the earliest white people to have shown up in Kansas. We've got all this history of Bleeding Kansas and John Brown."

As a New Englander, I needed to do a bit of reading to gain a better grasp of Dan's background. "Bleeding Kansas," it turns out, is the term used to describe a five-year period in the 1850s during which paramilitary guerrilla warfare was waged between pro-slavery and anti-slavery groups. This was a barbaric time in which abolitionist Kansans and gangs based in Missouri viciously fought with each other, sacking and pillaging towns.

---

[1] Scott Cacciola, "Yes, they are tall. No, they do not play basketball," *The New York Times*, March 21, 2023, https://www.nytimes.com/2023/03/21/sports/basketball/tall-basketball-march-madness.html.

Nowadays, the name John Brown evokes the folksong that Union soldiers marched to in the Civil War and which the singer Pete Seeger popularized again. The actual historical figure was inextricably involved in Bleeding Kansas, and he believed himself to have a "sacred obligation" to end slavery."[2] He led a small group of men, including his adult sons, on a series of raids against pro-slavery forces before being executed by hanging following an unsuccessful attempt to incite an insurrection at the Harper's Ferry (now West Virginia) federal armory.

In Kansas, the decision about slavery was to be made by a popular vote of the Territory's settlers, which would eventually determine whether to join the Union or Confederacy. The anti-slavery proponents—like John Brown—who opposed the institution on religious, philosophical, and humanitarian grounds, proved to be in the majority, and Kansas was officially admitted by Congress as a free state.

I am hardly unique in holding the oversimplistic belief that "in the quest for symbols of down-home, stand-pat, plainspoken, unvarnished, bedrock American goodness Kansas has everyone else beat."[3] But the origin story of Kansas does not exactly dovetail with it being a tranquil, rural place where Dorothy gratefully lazed about after returning from Oz and Clark Kent led a quiet boyhood with his adopted parents. Instead, according to a native Kansan, author Thomas Frank, there is a streak of weird that periodically surfaces: "The place has crawled with religious fanatics, crackpot demagogues, and alarming hybrids of the two . . . and Free Love to Prohibition, utopian communism to the John Birch Society—were embraced quickly and ardently." Both Dodge City and Abilene were justifiably famous for their murderous cowboys. In 1923, approximately 60,000 Kansans were Ku Klux Klan members and espoused that organization's virulent white supremacy, anti-Semitism, and anti-Catholicism.[4] In 1966, the Beat Generation godfather, Allen Ginsburg, used a Guggenheim fellowship to purchase a Volkswagen van and drive into Wichita with his boyfriend, Peter Orlovsky; there, he would compose and recite his masterpiece, the Wichita Vortex Sutra, to considerable acclaim and consternation.[5] Most recently, in August of 2022, politically red Kansas surprised the nation when a solid majority of voters soundly rejected a proposed state constitutional amendment that would have banned access to abortions.[6]

[2] Gamaliel Bradford, "John Brown," *The Atlantic Online*, accessed June 18, 2023, https://www.theatlantic.com/past/docs/issues/22nov/bradford.htm.

[3] Thomas Frank, *What's the Matter with Kansas* (New York: Henry Holt and Company, 2004).

[4] Ibid.

[5] "Wichita Vortex – A KPTS Documentary," PBS, accessed August 17, 2022, https://www.youtube.com/watch?v=9NeSJNi0xcM.

[6] Dylan Lysen, Laura Ziegler, and Blaise Mesa, "Voters in Kansas decide to keep abortion legal in the state, rejecting an amendment," NPR, accessed August 16, 2022, https://www.npr.org/sections/

As Dan recounted to me the details of his family's experiences during Bleeding Kansas, the anecdotes had a prophetic ring. I had a feeling they might prove to be important to his own saga, but I wouldn't realize the extent until later.

Jumping to more recent generations of Winters, Dan explained that his kin included largely conservative politicians, prosperous bankers, staid attorneys, and other respected members of the establishment. After watching his father and brother become state senators, Dan was clear, "I wouldn't run for office for a million dollars." He further clarified, "But I would work to get other people elected," and he campaigned for numerous candidates.

Members of the Winter clan have been community leaders who were especially quick and foresightful in recognizing entrepreneurial opportunities. Dan told me, "My grandfather coached football at Kansas State University for a while. Then he purchased several car dealerships, became the editor of the local newspaper, and operated three large cattle ranches in adjacent states." Dan's father, Wint, acquired several community banks, drilled for oil, and owned a successful Pizza Hut franchise in Mississippi. Aside from his political career, he was a rodeo cowboy and served as a district court judge. Kansas movers and shakers were regular visitors to the Winter home, and, as a child, Dan remembers opening a bathroom door to unexpectedly find "the bare bottom of [then Kansas US Senator] Bob Dole," who had just stepped out of the shower.

Because Wint was on the road a lot, Dan and his four siblings infrequently saw their father for more than a couple of days a week. To make up for his absence, the man would sometimes show up at the schoolroom door and boisterously yank the boys from the classroom. "Before I knew it," Dan cheerfully recalled, "I might find myself on Dad's light plane on route to Butte, Montana or Mobile, Alabama or Santa Fe, New Mexico or Saskatoon, Saskatchewan."

According to Dan, his father's side of the family is from English-German stock. A reunion was filled with "weirdly square-jawed guys who all seemed to look alike." In the photographs he sent me, it is evident that Dan has inherited this same facial feature. By contrast, he explained that, like much of the Kansas City population, his mother's people were Irish. "So, I grew up culturally Irish," he continued.

"Which means what?" I asked.

"Alcoholism," he instantly replied. "Plus speaking your mind, and loudly letting everybody know what you think and feel."

*****

2022-live-primary-election-race-results/2022/08/02/1115317596/kansas-voters-abortion-legal-reject-constitutional-amendment.

One advantage that comes with knowing you have an irreversible disease like Alzheimer's and will be taking your life is that you're in a great position to write your own obituary. Dan was no doubt broadly grinning when he composed the following lines that would eventually appear in his *Oregonian* announcement: "Flouting family tradition, Dan, was an average athlete. Nonetheless, he persisted. He was the kid riding the bench who cheered the loudest, and the one who was used as the blocking dummy in practice. As a senior, after he finally got a starting spot, the sports editor of the town paper responded with 'REALLY?' "[7]

More successful in scholastic and social pursuits than athletic ones, Dan was appointed the high school newspaper editor. Popular with his peers, he won the Rotary Club's Student of the Year award and was named the Homecoming King.

According to his brother-in-law, Steve Stingley, the self-proclaimed "pinnacle" of Dan's high school days came at the big football game. Before it began, Dan stood alone in the middle of the field. "Dressed in his red and white Cyclone football uniform, cheeks blackened under his eyes to prevent the glare of the bright lights, helmet tucked under his arm," Steve would write, "this tall and handsome young man sang the national anthem to the packed crowd. Later that same night, he would be the guy to crown the homecoming queen."

"It was a great feeling for me," Dan recalled. "I was the *shit*."

After majoring in journalism at the University of Kansas, Dan earned a bachelor of science degree and then began working his way up through the chain of command in the family-owned financial institutions. Dan became the president and CEO of a group of community banks located in eastern Kansas, Colorado, and New Mexico, and later he would be the chair of a small holding company that owned the banks. Dan eventually launched a self-financed venture in mortgage banking, but he would leave that position and be appointed Executive Director of the American Civil Liberties Union of Kansas and Western Missouri.

The administrative position at the ACLU allowed him to pursue a longstanding passion defending civil rights. To his delight, he might find himself mediating LGBTQ disputes in the morning and then laboring over abortion access in the afternoon. The next day could be spent entangled in knotty racial discrimination issues. Throughout this time, Dan lobbied legislative committees and did a lot of public advocacy speaking. He was especially proud to have served over a 10-year period as the treasurer for Planned Parenthood Great Plains.

Dan and his wife, Wynne, sent their children to a Catholic parochial school, but, on account of his involvement with Planned Parenthood, they were threatened by the local priest with excommunication. Labeled a "baby killer" by some members of the parish, Dan received an anonymous call from a man who

---

[7] "Daniel Patrick Winter obituary," *Oregonian*, accessed March 14, 2023, https://obits.oregonl ive.com/us/obituaries/oregon/name/daniel-winter-obituary?id=9278887.

said he intended to firebomb the Winter home and "watch it burn to the ground with your family in it."

Dan immediately reported the call to police, and four squad cars and a firetruck arrived at his doorstep to unsuccessfully scour the property for any signs of explosives. Some years later the man who had telephoned acknowledged what he did, apologized, and confessed to have been inebriated at the time.

But that wasn't Dan's only conflict over Catholic doctrine. "His disenchantment with the Church," according to John, "started in grade school when one of Dan's dogs died. Dan told the nun, who was his teacher, that 'at least he'd get to see the dog in heaven.' The nun declared to Dan, 'Dogs don't go to heaven because they don't have souls.' Even as a child, Dan knew this wasn't possible. Dogs were *nothing* but souls."

A friend would later report to me, "Like Dan, some of his kinfolk have held progressive opinions, but the family always resided in a state that has a highly conservative culture with only islands of liberalism. Dan's family was all about following the rules of white Republican, Kansas upper middle-class culture, and there was powerful pressure on him to march along with everyone else. The extended Winter clan was Kennedyesque . . . very privileged . . . a lot of money . . . really charming."

"So, how did you develop your progressive social beliefs," I asked Dan. "What made you passionate about social justice?"

He described his upbringing as one of five siblings raised in a small town situated between Lawrence and Kansas City. When he was 10 years old and his dad was running for the State Senate in Kansas as a moderate Republican, he learned Martin Luther King had been assassinated. The following morning, the entire family's attention was riveted by the television coverage. Dan remembers his mother objecting to the children being present and his father saying, "Of course, they need to watch." Later, his mom and dad called all the kids out to the backyard flagpole where they had a little ceremony in honor of MLK. First, they raised the flag, and then they silently lowered it to half staff.

"That night," Dan said, "I looked out the window of my bedroom and it appeared as if the house was ablaze. I woke everyone up. The fire department and the police were summoned, and they quickly arrived with sirens howling, only to discover that somebody had tried to burn a cross in the yard."

After everyone departed, the family would later find a note left in their mailbox by the perpetrator. It read, "Wint, I nearly shit my skivvies when I saw that you lowered your flag to half-mast after they killed that n****r."

"Jesus!" Dan exclaimed to me. "This is a tranquil, diminutive town of 10,000 people. A big bell went off in my brain." Dan's epiphany was, *Maybe there's a place for me to try to change all of that.*

5

On the surface, Dan's life—both childhood and adulthood—seemed enviable . . . that is, perhaps, except for the firebombing threat and the cross-burning. Apart from his academic and professional accomplishments, he met and married an extraordinary woman, had three lovely children, and they resided in an immaculate home situated in the outskirts of Kansas City, which he decorated with carefully curated mid-20th-century regional art. The kids attended private schools, and the couple were highly regarded philanthropists and mainstays of their community.

Catherine Frazee, professor emerita from the School of Disability Studies at Toronto Metropolitan University, has written about how little is known regarding "the impact of the experience of sudden vulnerability upon persons who have enjoyed social and material privilege and security."[1] She goes on to say, the "experience in Oregon and other jurisdictions with permissive approaches to physician-hastened death suggests that those who advocate for and actively pursue this option tend to cluster demographically in privileged social groups, prompting some to describe them as 'the three W's: white, wealthy and well-educated.'"

Dan could certainly claim full membership in the three W's. Professor Frazee might have pointed out that as a healthy, able-bodied man who had enjoyed a lifetime of physical vigor and social privilege, he likely felt that having to depend on others all day long would be intolerable.

The first of the W's deserves particular attention because race, ethnicity, and culture have made marked impacts on advance care planning and palliative care

[1] Catherine Frazee, "'The vulnerable': Who are they?," Canadian Virtual Hospice, accessed December 15, 2022, https://www.virtualhospice.ca/en_US/Main+Site+Navigation/Home/For+Professionals/For+Professionals/The+Exchange/Current/%E2%80%9CThe+Vulnerable%E2%80%9D_+Who+Are+They_.aspx.

in Western and Eastern cultures.[2-4] For example, an examination of bereaved family members where the deceased were 70 and older found that white patients were significantly more likely to have discussed treatment preferences than Black patients, designated a durable power of attorney for healthcare, and completed a living will.[5] Treatment decisions for Black patients were purportedly based on a desire to provide "all care possible in order to prolong life," in contrast to treat- ment decisions for white patients, which were more likely to involve "limiting care in certain situations" and "withholding treatment before death."

In another study, Black and white adults aged 65 and older receiving primary care treatment were surveyed on advance care planning, beliefs about dying, and attitudes regarding hospice care.[6] Black patients were again less likely than white subjects to have completed an advance directive, and they had less favorable beliefs about hospice treatment. They were more likely to want aggressive care at the end of life, have spiritual beliefs that conflict with the goals of palliative med- icine, express discomfort discussing death, and mistrust the healthcare system.

Also of interest is an older study that compared the attitudes of Black versus white physicians regarding end-of-life decision-making.[7] Doctors were asked about their own preferences if they theoretically sustained brain damage and were not terminally ill—a scenario comparable to what Dan was experiencing. Under that circumstance, the majority of all physicians did not want aggressive treatment; however, Black physicians were five times more likely than white physicians to request treatments, which included cardiopulmonary resuscita- tion, mechanical ventilation, and/or artificial feeding. In this hypothetical, white physicians were twice as likely as Black physicians to want medical aid in dying for themselves.

[2] Jack Pun, James C. H. Chow, Leslie Fok, and Ka Man Cheung, "Role of patients' family members in end-of-life communication: An integrative review," *BMJ Open* 13, no. 2 (February 2023): e067304, doi: 10.1136/bmjopen-2022-067304. PMID: 36810181; PMCID: PMC9945016.

[3] Zhongyi Fan, Liyan Chen, Limin Meng, et al., "Preference of cancer patients and family members regarding delivery of bad news and differences in clinical practice among medical staff," *Support Care Cancer* 27, no. 2 (February 2019): 583–589, doi: 10.1007/s00520-018-4348-1.

[4] K. W. Bowman and P. A. Singer, "Chinese seniors' perspectives on end-of-life decisions," *Social Science and Medicine* 53, no. 4 (August 2001): 455–464, doi: 10.1016/s0277-9536(00)00348.

[5] F. P. Hopp and S. A. Duffy, "Racial variations in end-of-life care," *Journal of the American Geriatric Society* 48, no. 6 (June 2000): 658–663, doi: 10.1111/j.1532-5415.2000.tb04724.x.

[6] Kimberly S. Johnson, Maragatha Kuchibhatla, and James A. Tulsky, "What explains ra- cial differences in the use of advance directives and attitudes toward hospice care?," *Journal of the American Geriatric Society* 56, no. 10 (October 2008): 1953–1958, https://doi.org/10.1111/ j.1532-5415.2008.01919.x

[7] Eric W. Mebane, Roy F. Oman, Leo T. Kroonen, and Mary K. Goldstein, "The influence of phy- sician race, age, and gender on physician attitudes toward advance care directives and preferences for end-of-life decision-making," *Journal of the American Geriatric Society* 47, no. 5 (May 1999): 579– 591, doi: 10.1111/j.1532-5415.1999.tb02573.x. PMID: 10323652.

Incidentally, "terminal" is defined as being an irreversible or incurable disease condition that results in death within the foreseeable future; however, although no consensus on the exact time frame exists and the survival duration varies within the U.S. Federal Code, many palliative care practitioners and some American assisted dying laws have settled on a 6 month or less duration. This is based on the arbitrary definition used to determine hospice eligibility.

I connected with Dr. LaVera Crawley, a vice president of pastoral and spiritual care at CommonSpirit Health System, to elicit her further reflections on end-of-life care differences and disparities between white and Black Americans. Dr. Crawley has previously written that the crux of the issue is often misrepresented by the suggestion that the onus is on patients to trust their providers. Instead, she explained to me (email May 17, 2023) that prior behaviors on the part of clinicians toward Black patients have repetitively and historically constituted "breaches of trust and thereby reduce the chance that those patients will go on to place unearned trust in future providers."[8]

The themes that Dr. Crawley illuminated, along with her coauthor, Alan Elbaum, are that "the struggle of African Americans for the right to exist, the injustice of premature Black deaths, and the experience of health systems-level and provider-level discrimination—underlie the perspective that death is a struggle to be overcome. While not every African American patient has had these experiences or holds these perspectives, the inequities are, nevertheless, part of the cultural narrative within the African American community."[9]

All told, the cultural issues in end-of-life decision-making—be they among Blacks, Hispanics, Asians, and Indigenous people, or among those who are part of religious communities, or those who self-identify as being members of the military, having disabilities, and other special populations, are likely to be exceedingly different from that of individuals, like Dan, who hailed from the three W's.[10] Likewise, throw into the mix the varying regional and national belief sets—Australians as a group have different views from Germans, who have different views from the English, Chinese, Saudis, or Canadians—and it all seems to overwhelming for us to come to terms with our common mortality.

*****

[8] LaVera Crawley, David Ahn, and Marilyn Winkleby, "Perceived medical discrimination and cancer screening behaviors of racial and ethnic minority adults," *Cancer Epidemiology Biomarkers & Prevention* 17, no. 8 (August 2008): 1937–1944, https://doi.org/10.1158/1055-9965.

[9] Alan Elbaum and Lavera Crawley, "Race and physician-assisted death: Do Black lives matter?," in Sheldon Rubenfeld and Daniel Sulmasy (eds.), *Physician Assisted Suicide and Euthanasia Before, During and After the Third Reich* (Lanham, MD, Rowman & Littlefield, 2020).

[10] Kathryn L. Braun, James H. Pietsch, Patricia L. Blanchette, *Cultural Issues in End-of-Life Decision Makin* (Thousand Oaks, CA: Sage, 2000).

Although I, too, am a member of the three W's, I was struck by the considerable dissimilarities between Dan and me. Kansas? Philanthropy? A senator for a father? A memory mirror decorated with allusions to the family-owned ranches where the young Dan worked alongside rough-and-tumble cowboys? A mother who donated money for a Catholic chapel? Keepsakes that included selections of poetry and a photograph of a ballet star?

Perhaps the biggest differences between us, however, lay hidden, carefully tucked beneath the surface. To begin, Dan was gay.

Willie Nelson may have been gently poking fun when he recorded Ned Sublette's song, "Cowboys Are Frequently, Secretly Fond of Each Other," but there was nothing humorous about Dan's situation out there on the prairie.[11] In the hypermasculine Kansas world in which he was raised, as a member of a family of prominent politicians, star athletes, and community leaders, such things weren't acknowledged to exist. The poet Allen Ginsberg may have swept through Kansas with his male partner when Dan was eight years old, but that wasn't a topic of conversation at the Winter family table.

Currently, 7% of Americans self-identify as gay, lesbian, bisexual, transgender, or something other than heterosexual, which is double the percentage from just 10 years earlier.[12] When Dan was a youngster, a scion of the Winter clan simply could not be homosexual. If lowering their flag to honor Martin Luther King, Jr. provoked outrage among some townsfolk, the community's reaction to any declaration regarding sexuality could barely be imagined.

Although he felt "different" from an early age, and in retrospect is convinced that his father recognized he was gay and worried about how it would impact his life, Dan's first homosexual experience didn't take place until age 42.

"When that happened, I was deeply shaken," he would later confide to his brother-in-law, Steve Stingley. "He was an acquaintance from the gym, and I had begun to have this niggling feeling that my sexual identity needed to be dealt with. I couldn't deny that I was having sexual thoughts about men. . . . I realized I'm gay, and what I mean by gay is I'm nearly a 10 on the spectrum of being gay. If I didn't start telling the truth to myself, I would explode."

Dan told Steve, "It became a question less about sex than identity. I began to realize I had an issue, and this wasn't going to go away."

[11] Emily Mack, "Willie Nelson recorded a famous gay cowboy song," Wide Open Country, accessed August 20, 2022, https://www.wideopencountry.com/cowboys-are-frequently-secretly-fond-of-eachother/.

[12] Jeffrey Jones, "LGBT identification in U.S. ticks up to 7.1%," Gallup, accessed August 17, 2022, https://news.gallup.com/poll/389792/lgbt-identification-ticks-up.aspx?campaign_id=39&emc=edit_ty_20220429&instance_id=59914&nl=opinion-today&regi_id=63340269&segment_id=90741&te=1&user_id=895343099129dcd1f95fa65a5a136796.

But homosexuality wasn't the only difference between him and me, nor was it the primary source of his distress.

Dan had been groomed by a football coach who, despite the boy's clumsiness on the gridiron, showered him with praise and made him feel exceptional. Having come from a family of accomplished competitors, the compliments were especially meaningful. Dan was 15 and a sophomore in high school when the man cornered him in his office and brutally assaulted and raped him. For many days, the boy secretly threw away pairs of his blood-stained underpants. Kept tightly under wraps, the attack was a source of indelible shame. Afterward, the memory of the trauma always bubbled beneath his thoughts, threatening to erupt at any moment. Dan had flashbacks consisting of vivid monochromatic black-and-white images of the attack, and they played over and over and over again in a repetitive loop.

The rape ripped him from his sheltered childhood and left the boy convinced that everyone in town was somehow aware he had been violated. Like most victims of trauma, he unfairly questioned his responsibility for what occurred. After the abuse, there was a layer of seriousness about Dan's life that had never been there before, and internally he became both stronger and much bleaker. He developed an impulsive tendency that manifested itself in a variety of maladaptive behaviors.

Dan felt guilty and different from his peers, which led him to begin regularly drinking. Alcohol served as an escape from reality and a means to bond with the other kids who drank. The boy also compensated by compulsively seeking to make people feel comfortable in his presence. Becoming well-liked and popular—it was no accident that he was elected to be the Homecoming King—helped salve but could not erase his shame and embarrassment.

Furthermore, athletic injuries—it's not a great idea to be a tackle dummy—required three corrective orthopedic back surgeries, and these led him to develop an addiction to prescription pain medications. According to John, "Dan went through the first half of his life with one hand wrapped around a bottle of vodka," but after the surgical procedures, he also walked about with a whole bunch of pills rattling in his pockets. According to one account, the polysubstance abuse ceased only after he totaled his prized, supercharged Jaguar XJ and spent a night in the drunk tank.

For decades, Dan vigilantly censored his opinions and mostly concealed the drinking and other pathological behaviors. "I tried in all ways to appear perfect," he told me, and, well into his 40s, Dan mostly succeeded. But one cannot overestimate the soul-crushing damage that childhood sexual abuse had wrought.

As Dan remembers it, around 2005, he was finally forced to admit, "that my life was kind of coming apart in the way lives come apart for advantaged people like me." Dan *wasn't* facing unemployment, homelessness, criminal charges, or hunger. Rather, "I didn't know what I wanted to do next. . . . I didn't know which direction to take my life, personally, professionally, or financially. My back injuries were acting up, and my wife and I were planning a divorce and talking about how to inform the kids that I was gay."

Around the same time, he and his sister listened to a radio news broadcast about a clergy sexual abuse case. She must have seen something in his face because she asked him point-blank whether he'd ever been abused. His first reaction was to deny it. Several hours later, he confessed the truth to her.

And, within the next few months, he began to widely disclose his secrets . . . all of his secrets.

With the help of "lots of psychotherapy," Dan determinedly rebounded after many years of silent torture and started to speak up. His victimization and anguish were transformed into righteous indignation, and he realized that the act of telling—the catharsis—contributed to his healing.

While many abuse survivors or alcoholics feel compelled to remain quiet about their experiences or share them only with close friends and other survivors, Dan believed both the Winter family and their extended community needed to fully hear about what had happened. He would later allow the story to be posted online—where I read it—and he did not hesitate from repeatedly talking to family and friends about the abuse and addictions.

He co-founded a group called the Kansas City Anti-Violence Coalition that was invited to local schools to talk about sexual abuse. The first time he spoke publicly about being assaulted was at a fundraising event for the coalition.

"Sexual abuse is very democratic," Dan explained to the audience. "Rich kids, poor kids—there is no one who is really safe from it. But it's a very tough subject to talk about."

As he became more comfortable speaking, Dan resolved to be an authentic self—capable of naming his traumas, challenging societal taboos, and fearlessly expressing his preferences. He decided that an honest, open life was infinitely preferable to remaining inhibited and mute.

Dan sat down with his wife, Wynne (yes, her name was Wynne, his father's nickname was Wint, and Winter was everyone's surname) to talk about their marriage and about being a gay man. Dan arrived at an arrangement with his spouse that allowed them to remain together until the children were older. In 2006, the couple agreed to separate, and they were divorced two years later. Although his work at the ACLU was deeply satisfying and Dan was financially comfortable, following a lifetime in Kansas he was ready to risk making a move. In 2011, he retired from the ACLU and purchased a condominium 1,800 miles away in Portland, Oregon.

Dan freely admitted that Wynne and their two sons and daughter were justifiably enraged at him. He had put them through hell, and he understood there was a large debt due for his many indiscretions. Dan explained, "They felt swindled. They felt like we had created something that wasn't real." In the face of their bitterness, for many years he persisted in trying to establish new, reparative relationships. Dan was desperate to earn back their love, and he was prepared to allow the process to take as long as was necessary.

When I spoke with Jack, his 31-year-old son, a sports journalist who also moved to Portland, he said (October 18, 2020), "Our relationship is now arguably as good as it's ever been in my life. We're as close as we've ever been." He characterized his father as having been a selfish narcissist. It had taken a lot of time, but Jack now felt comfortable saying, "My dad really does love me and my siblings and my mom in the best way he can."

While I realized this wasn't exactly a full-throated endorsement, Jack wistfully concluded, "Whenever I'm looking back on all this, in however many years, I think it will be a point of solace."

A major factor in Dan's decision to settle in Oregon was the state's Death with Dignity Act, which he felt was a socially responsible law that spoke exceedingly well for Oregonians. Enacted in 1997 after two referendums, this was America's first medical aid in dying statute. It was designed to allow suffering, terminally ill people to accelerate their deaths with the participation of a physician. At first, the Winter family thought the importance Dan accorded to controlling death was a bit bizarre. But ultimately, they came to respect his opinion, and it allowed them to crystalize their own varied end-of-life positions.

Dan's observations about his father's drawn-out descent into Alzheimer's, along with his support of autonomy and the right-to-die movement, all served as bridges between him and me. From the beginning of our relationship, Dan understood that although we were allies, he oversaw the narrative. My role would be to transcribe his story and to faithfully respect the course that he set— wherever it led.

6

In 2011, John David Forsgren was not looking to establish a new relationship when he found himself sitting alongside Dan at a small dinner gathering convened by Pauline and Drew Lewis in their Portland apartment. Yet the attraction and chemistry between the two men was magical; 3 months later, they moved in together. According to John, "A lesbian friend said it was a very lesbian thing to do—the joke being that the moving van comes at the first date."

The relationship, which began when John was 60 and Dan 52, worked in good measure because neither man believed in bottling things up. According to John, "There is a level of honesty and eagerness to continue to learn in Dan that is extremely appealing. He's smart in the ways that I'm not. He's funny. He makes me laugh. After some pretty dark years, Dan has allowed me to become my better self."

"Things just happened," John said. "We were powerless. I've loved several different kinds of men and learned to see love expressed differently. Dan is very comfortable saying he loves me and describing why, and that's pretty great."

John and Dan were also in agreement that "having both been around the block a few times and falling in love late in life, you're less concerned about being right about everything."

In May of 2014, same-sex marriage was legalized in Oregon, and the two men heard the news while vacationing in New York City. While they hardly thought of themselves as "foolish romantics," they got engaged the same night.

John explained, "However, by the time we got around to trying to find a judge to marry us, every gay and lesbian couple in the Portland metro area had already reserved their time. Dan knew that the communications director at the local ACLU office was a Universal Life Church minister. Several weeks later, she agreed to marry us in her office. We told her that we just wanted to bring our two witnesses for a 'service.' But upon our arrival, we were led into the conference room, which had been decorated with streamers, a table with a cake and bottles of sparkling apple juice, and rows of chairs facing the front. Apparently, the staff wanted to attend.

"In the end, we had to be Grinches and tell them that we couldn't let family and friends know this was happening, so getting married in front of a room full of strangers didn't seem quite right. They understood, and we were wed with just our two witnesses. There was a celebration a couple of months later at what was then our new home; in attendance were a couple of hundred friends and family, including several of the ACLU staff. Happy times. . . ."

John was one of four siblings raised in a small, highly conservative Oregon town. His father was a medical internist, his mother a nurse, and "they were socially liberal and very direct about life and disease, illness and death."

At age 6, John began to identify with a few other boys whom he later understood to be homosexual. A perennial outsider whose hair inexplicably developed a prominent white streak when he was in high school, he characterized himself as being an "observer of American culture, rather than a participant."

John was a teenager when the Stonewall uprising took place in 1969. He was keenly aware of demonstrations by the gay community, but "it was something that I never discussed with anybody. Nor did I reveal having seen any articles in the newspaper or pictures in *Life Magazine*," he told me. "I certainly remember seeing those black-and-white photos of men being arrested . . . and I also vividly recall Liberace. Those were sum total of the gay men that I was exposed to. There was nothing that was grounding for me . . . nothing that I could recognize or move toward. However, I watched the gay rights movement grow and develop in the '70s."

As a youth, John played piano, sang in choirs, and eventually became a gym rat in order to deal with back pain and also stay thin. After college, he acquired a degree in architecture and joined a large firm, where he remained until the recession crippled the industry. John then supported himself as an interior designer and artist.

In the spring of 1981, he had a transformative experience when he found a magazine piece about a novel medical syndrome that would soon come to be called HIV/AIDS. At the time, he had a brand-new roommate who moved to Portland from Los Angeles. "While I was reading this article in my kitchen about these weird symptoms that were showing up, um, Chris was upstairs having most of them. So, for me, the disease was never abstract."

When acquired immunodeficiency syndrome (AIDS) spread through Oregon, ravaging every corner of the state, John got to see the darkest side of humanity and of American medicine. Nationally, from 1981 through 1990, more than 100,000 deaths were reported to the Centers for Disease Control.[1] In 1987,

---

[1] "Current trends mortality attributable to HIV infection/AIDS: United States, 1981–1990," *MMWR Weekly*, CDC, accessed August 18, 2022, https://www.cdc.gov/mmwr/preview/mmwrh

there were 10,000 deaths in New York City alone.[2] By 1989, AIDS was estimated to be the second leading cause of death in the country among men 25–44 years of age, surpassing cancer, suicide, cardiac disease, and homicide. The federal government responded with almost total indifference, and it would be years before a president would publicly utter the word "AIDS." Little research was performed to ascertain the cause or explore treatments, and what existed was shamefully underfunded. About half of Americans who contracted the virus during that period died of an HIV/AIDS-related condition within 2 years.

As gay men became ill, they turned to their parents and siblings for support. Unfortunately, many of those families rejected and abandoned their sons and brothers, experiencing the illness as a source of unbearable embarrassment. Weakened, disfigured, and dying from the disease, these young men were admitted to large municipal and small community hospitals. Meal trays would frequently be left on the floor outside of their rooms by worried staff, and they were only brought inside by other gay men, like John, who came for visits.

Change only began after Diana, Princess of Wales, went to the London Middlesex Hospital. In front of the world's media, she shook the hand of a man dying from AIDS and declared, "HIV does not make people dangerous to know. So, you can shake their hand and give them a hug. Heaven knows they need it."[3] Her gesture challenged the commonly held belief that HIV or AIDS could be transmitted by touch.

In a subsequent speech, she said: "AIDS is no respecter of color, class, or creed. Nor does it hold international boundaries in high regard. All too soon, we will all know someone with AIDS: a brother, sister, mother, father, son, or daughter could be next. How will we treat them? With compassion and care? Or fear and rejection?"[4]

Even when families supported their loved ones along every inch of the journey, it was horrible. Right-to-die executive Peg Sandeen wrote to me (March 3, 2023): "To have the most basic of dignities stripped from you at the end of your life is devastating. My husband John underwent a devastating decline as

tml/00001880.htm#:~:text=From%201981%20through%201990%2C%20100%2C777,deaths%20were%20reported%20during%201990.

[2] Matt Flegenheimer and Rosa Goldensohn, "The secrets Ed Koch carried," *The New York Times*, accessed August 20, 2022, https://www.nytimes.com/2022/05/07/nyregion/ed-koch-gay-secrets.html?campaign_id=9&emc=edit_nn_20220508&instance_id=60799&nl=the-morning&regi_id=122063637&segment_id=91650&te=1&user_id=08f1f0033c8df71cd58b9f516c748586.

[3] Josh Milton, "Princess Diana changed how the world saw HIV and AIDS with one simple but profound gesture," PinkNews, August 31, 2022, https://www.pinknews.co.uk/2022/08/31/princess-diana-hiv-aids/.

[4] "Princess Diana speaks about AIDS," YouTube, accessed August 31, 2022, https://www.youtube.com/watch?v=UAvvM12eMQM.

he died following an HIV diagnosis while experiencing substantial symptoms of AIDS-related dementia. This was in the 1990s, and John had few choices at the end of his life. Medical assistance in dying (MAiD) wasn't legal anywhere in the country; voluntarily stopping eating and drinking wasn't part of the conversation. AIDS sufferers whispered about taking overdoses; the avoidance or withdrawal of life-prolonging medical treatments and making use of palliative sedation were just beginning to be considered."

Dr. Shannon Mazur, a psycho-oncologist and bioethicist from Yale Smilow Cancer Hospital, told me (March 25, 2023) that the latter is "a measure of last resort when conventional therapies have been unsuccessful at providing symptom relief, and medications are given to the patient to induce a state of continuous decreased or absent awareness (unconsciousness)."[5] Palliative sedation is most frequently done in a hospital setting, although it can theoretically be performed in a care facility or home, and the medications can be provided subcutaneously (under the skin), rectally, or intravenously.[6-9] Although palliative sedation is common in European countries and legal in all 50 US states, many large American medical centers, including hers, still lack a formal policy and clinical protocol to meet the needs of patients for palliative care and to address clinician concerns surrounding legal liability.[10]

Peg Sandeen explained that after her husband died, "I became a social worker and a political activist because I wanted to give others what I couldn't give my beloved husband—a choice to retain the same dignity in death that he had while healthy."

---

[5] Patricia Claessens, Johan Menten, Paul Schotsmans, and Bert Broeckaert, "Palliative sedation: A review of the research literature," *Journal of Pain and Symptom Management* 36, no. 3 (September 2008): 310–333, doi: 10.1016/j.jpainsymman.2007.10.004. Epub 2008 Jul 25. PMID: 18657380.

[6] Andrew Billings and Susan D. Block, "Slow euthanasia," *Journal of Palliative Care* 12, no. 4 (December 1996): 21–30, doi:10.1177/082585979601200404.

[7] Judith Setla and Silviu Valeriu Pasniciuc, "Home palliative sedation using phenobarbital suppositories: Time to death, patient characteristics, and administration protocol," *American Journal of Hospice and Palliative Care* 36, no. 10 (October 2019): 871–876, doi: 10.1177/1049909119839695. Epub 2019 Apr 4. PMID: 30947512.

[8] Alexander de Graeff and Mervyn Dean, "Palliative sedation therapy in the last weeks of life: A literature review and recommendations for standards," *Journal of Palliative Medicine* 10, no. 1 (February 2007): 67–85, doi: 10.1089/jpm.2006.0139.

[9] Eva Schildmann and Jan Schildmann, "Palliative sedation therapy: A systematic literature review and critical appraisal of available guidance on indication and decision making," *Journal of Palliative Medicine* 17, no. 5 (May 2014): 601–611, doi: 10.1089/jpm.2013.0511.

[10] Ronald R. Cranford and Raymond Gensinger, "Hospital policy on terminal sedation and euthanasia," *HEC Forum* 14, no. 3 (2002): 259–264, https://www.proquest.com/scholarly-journals/hospital-policy-on-terminal-sedation-euthanasia/docview/220118771/se-2.

In 1985, John Forsgren tested positive for HIV, but, unlike almost everyone else in his circle, John never came down with AIDS. Nevertheless, he went home convinced that he was going to die. After "coming out" during his 10th high school reunion, unlike many of his friends, he had been warmly embraced by his parents. Now, when John rejoined his mother, father, and younger sister, the family had just returned to Oregon after having spent much of 1974–1975 running two poverty medical practices in rural South Vietnam. John explained that they were trying "to make up for what our government was doing in the war."

Throughout much of the 1980s and 1990s, John transformed himself into an AIDS activist. He was determined to fight for his community's lives and basic rights. In Portland, he served on the board of a local AIDS education and fundraising organization within the art community. During this period, John was convinced that it was only a matter of time before he developed the syndrome. "It was a point in my life," he explained, "when it wasn't always easy to be optimistic."

Around 1996–1997, the first effective therapies became available; 14 years before he met Dan, John began taking the retroviral medication cocktail. "In about 3 weeks, I realized that I was a different person. Wow! I had my strength back, plus I felt a kernel of hope."

If one thinks AIDS is merely a historical artifact, it is worth noting that HIV is still killing in gargantuan numbers around the world. So far, it has ended the lives of some 40 million people—more than from the COVID pandemic.[11] As many as *650,000 of those deaths occurred in 2021 alone.*[12] It has also long ceased to be a "gay disease."

To his credit, George W. Bush started the President's Emergency Plan for AIDS Relief, or PEPFAR, a global effort to turn the tide of the HIV/AIDS pandemic.[13] January 28, 2023, was the 20th anniversary of the program, and the U.S. government has invested more than $100 billion—the largest commitment by any nation to address a single disease in history. PEPFAR is estimated to have so far saved 25 million lives worldwide.

But, back in 1996, while John felt physically stabilized, he began to mourn and grieve the cumulative deaths of his friends. How many? Back in 1989, he had ceased counting after reaching 100. "I fell completely under the seductive

---

[11] "Is the end of AIDS in sight? The virus can be brought under control, but it's complicated," *The Economist*, September 17, 2023, accessed September 18, 2023.

[12] "Despite setbacks, HIV can be beaten," *The Economist*, accessed August 30, 2022, https://www.economist.com/science-and-technology/2022/08/02/despite-setbacks-hiv-can-be-beaten.

[13] "The United States President's Emergency Plan for AIDS Relief," U.S. Department of State, accessed March 20, 2023, https://www.state.gov/pepfar/#:~:text=Through%20PEPFAR%2C%20the%20U.S.%20government,global%20HIV%2FAIDS%20pandemic%20in.

nature of depression," he realized, and John's vibrancy, his ability to experience joy, and his pleasure in expressing himself through art were each dampened. While the effects of posttraumatic stress disorder and clinical depression had lifted when he met Dan, the experience was not one that could be entirely repressed or forgotten.

My colleague, Dr. James Rundell, a professor of psychiatry at Louisiana State University School of Medicine in Shreveport, felt his pulse quicken as he read this segment of the story (August 28, 2022). He wrote me, "Having dodged a bullet changes almost everyone's view towards our eventual mortality."

*****

When Dan and John met, the former was not only adjusting to having left his life in Kansas and moving to Portland, he was also enmeshed in what became an intensive multiyear campaign to reestablish a loving relationship with his children and ex-wife, Wynne. Each of them sought to determine whether the "new Dan" could be trusted. "For years my sons and daughter didn't speak to me," he explained with remorse. "It was not because of my sexuality, but because they were so very disappointed that their family wasn't what they thought it was." Dan regretted the many instances in which he had been duplicitous and unreliable.

Then the Sandusky scandal erupted and further complicated matters.[14]

Jerry Sandusky, a celebrated college football coach from Pennsylvania State University, was arrested and charged with 52 counts involving the abuse of young boys. Indicted, tried, and found guilty, the media bombardment was nonstop.

According to John, Dan reacted to the frenzy over the story "physically, like he'd gotten a gut punch . . . it seemed to knock all the air out of him." Dan was retraumatized as more and more graphic testimony was broadcast about the celebrity coach, and every mention of the case evoked memories of his own rape.

Dan sought relief by attending individual psychotherapy as well as participating in an organization called 1in6 and its online support group for male survivors of sexual assault.[15] As part of their Bristlecone Project, he agreed to have his own story posted. Although Dan did not formally accuse the coach who abused him in childhood, nor did he seek his punishment or contrition, the man was later "run out of town in the dark of night." According to John, "Dan suspected this was quietly orchestrated by the father of another boy he had abused."

In time, Dan was able to make excellent use of therapy. He was no longer drinking and using pain medications when he came to Portland. With John's

---

[14] "Penn State child sex abuse scandal," Wikipedia, accessed August 19, 2022, https://en.wikipedia.org/wiki/Penn_State_child_sex_abuse_scandal.

[15] Home page, 1in6, accessed August 20, 2022, https://1in6.org/.

help, he began to integrate himself into Portland society, joining philanthropic and social justice organizations, as well as exploring the local art scene. John and he carved out a satisfying life for themselves—one in which they acquired numerous friends who appreciated that the couple knew how to laugh and enjoy themselves but could also be depended upon to sensitively assist those who were in need. The two men were recognized to be *givers* and not *takers*.

In the meantime, Dan's father continued to be pummeled by Alzheimer's disease.

Before Wint was finally admitted to a specialized nursing facility, and while he was still capable of being managed at home by his wife, Dan and John came for a visit. Arriving at the house in Kansas, John couldn't help but observe that Wint no longer looked like a former state senator—a position he held for three terms. The Winter patriarch was aimlessly walking amidst the backyard garden's autumn foliage, picking up and carefully examining individual oak leaves. He would then set one down and reach over and clasp another, gazing at it in wonder like it was the first leaf he'd ever seen.

John explained to me that Wint "was wearing an overcoat, a pair of shoes without socks, and no trousers." The elderly man neither recognized nor acknowledged Dan and John's presence. He had never previously discussed his wishes regarding terminal care preferences, and, if he had any opinions, he was now entirely incapable of putting them into words. Dan and John found the visit to be emotionally devastating.

7

Several years earlier, Dan and I each separately stumbled upon an article that was published in *The New York Times Magazine*, "The last day of her life."[1] Robin Marantz Henig's piece began by describing how, in May of 2009, 64-year-old Dr. Sandra Bem watched a television documentary called "The Alzheimer's Project."[2]

In the 1960s, Sandy and her husband, Daryl, were celebrated as pioneering psychologists for the cause of gender equality. The two of them collaborated in developing the Bem Sex-Role Inventory, which was a psychological instrument based on an appreciation that every individual exhibits in varying degrees both male and female characteristics.[3] The Bems had become academic celebrities who contributed to changing America's clichés regarding the roles men and women could perform at work and home.

During the previous 2 years, Sandy had been having difficulty remembering names of people and had also been mixing up similar sounding words. The television broadcast crystalized for her the unpleasant possibility that she might have a dementia.

While researching my previous book, I contacted Daryl and some of their friends. Sandy was portrayed in these interviews as having been observant, sincere, compassionate, and a veritable junky for learning new things. She was loveable, but also occasionally irascible, tactless, and off-putting. The psychologist

[1] R. M. Henig, "The last day of her life," May 14, 2015, accessed August 25, 2022, https://www.nytimes.com/2015/05/17/magazine/the-last-day-of-her-life.html.

[2] "The Alzheimer's Project," HBO, accessed August 25, 2022, https://www.hbo.com/the-alzheimer-s-project.

[3] Carol J. Auster, "Bem Sex-Role Inventory," in Virgil Zeigler-Hill and Todd K Shackelford (eds.), *Encyclopedia of Personality and Individual Differences* (Cham: Springer), accessed August 25, 2022, https://doi.org/10.1007/978-3-319-24612-3_1207. 2020.

stood only 4′ 9″ tall, and, according to Henig, was "a tiny, little unprepossessing thing, who mainly wore jeans and work shirts."

Sandy had been an undergraduate when she met Daryl, who exclaimed on their first date, "I'm from Colorado, and I'm a stage magician, and I'm predominantly gay." During our interview, Daryl laughed uproariously while telling me that Sandy's immediate response was, "I don't think I've ever known anyone from Colorado."

They married 4 months later and had a son and a daughter. The Bems amicably separated when the children were 17 and 19; however, the couple continued to live just a few blocks away from each other. They remained the best of friends.

Karen Daschiff Gilovich, a neighbor and member of Sandy's inner circle, told me (March 20, 2009) that she was "unfettered by convention."

"It wasn't a shtick," Gilovich emphasized. "She was a powerful presence . . . unique. I remember one time she said, 'So, okay, why is it wrong for adults to have sex with children?'

"I was a psychotherapist specializing in child sexual abuse! I looked at her to see if she was kidding. But she was like, 'No, no, let's just not make any assumptions. Let's just break this down.' And so, I just thought, Okay, this is Sandy being Sandy."

On the lecture circuit, Sandy and Daryl proudly described how they refrained from discouraging their son from wearing pink barrettes to kindergarten, and how each day they intentionally drove their daughter past the same construction site. They thought it was important for her to see the woman clad in a hardhat who was a regular member of the crew.

One month after watching the documentary on Alzheimer's, Daryl drove Sandy from their home in Ithaca, New York, to the University of Rochester Medical Center for cognitive testing by a neuropsychologist. The clinician offered a preliminary diagnosis: amnestic mild cognitive impairment (MCI).[4] Sandy was relieved at hearing the word, "mild," until she saw the look on his face.

MCI is a clinical classification stage that resides between the expected cognitive decline of normal aging and the more serious deterioration associated with dementia.[5] It is manifested by memory, language, and judgment errors that

---

[4] Dana G. Smith, "What Is Mild Cognitive Impairment, and How Is It Diagnosed?," February 6, 2024, accessed February 9, 2024. https://www.nytimes.com/2024/02/06/well/mind/mild-cognitive-impairment-diagnosis.html?campaign_id=18&emc=edit_hh_20240208&instance_id=114688&nl=well&regi_id=63340269&segment_id=157702&te=1&user_id=895343099129dcd1f95fa65a5a136796

[5] Reisa A. Sperling, Paul S. Aisen, Laurel A. Beckett, et al., "Toward defining the preclinical stages of Alzheimer's disease: Recommendations from the National Institute on Aging-Alzheimer's Association workgroups on diagnostic guidelines for Alzheimer's disease," *Alzheimers Dement* 7, no. 3 (May 2011): 280–292, https://doi.org/10.1016/j.jalz.2011.03.003.

are more evident to the individual and to her family than would be normal age-related changes.[6,7] MCI can be broken down into either two or four different types based on the thinking skills that are affected: amnestic MCI (which primarily affects memory) and non-amnestic MCI (which affects the other cognitive abilities).[8,9] Research suggests that amnestic MCI is about twice as common as the non-amnestic type. According to the Alzheimer's Association, 15–20% of people aged 65 or older have MCI,[10] while a new study using nationally representative data has pegged the prevalence at 22%.[11] Depending on the sample and clinical criteria, the annual progression of people with amnestic MCI to Alzheimer's disease or another type of dementia varies between 4% and 17%; the majority receive a dementia diagnosis within 10 years.[12,13]

The neuropsychologist tried to soften his pronouncement by emphasizing that some people with MCI never get worse and a small number improve. But he also said, "I know your work, Dr. Bem, and I'm so sorry this has happened to you."

[6] D. A. Bennett, J. A. Schneider, J. L. Bienias, D. A. Evans, and R. S. Wilson, "Mild cognitive impairment is related to Alzheimer disease pathology and cerebral infarctions," *Neurology* 64, no. 5 (March 2005): 834–841, https://doi.org/10.1212/01.WNL.0000152982.47274.9E.

[7] B. Winblad, K. Palmer, M. Kivipelto, et al., "Mild cognitive impairment: Beyond controversies, towards a consensus: Report of the International Working Group on Mild Cognitive Impairment," *Journal of Internal Medicine* 256, no. 3 (September 2004):240–246, https://doi.org/10.1111/j.1365-2796.2004.01380.x.

[8] "Mild cognitive impairment (MCI)," Dementia Australia, accessed May 30, 2023, https://www.dementia.org.au/sites/default/files/helpsheets/Helpsheet-OtherInformation01-MildCognitiveImpairment_english.pdf.

[9] A. Busse, A. Hensel, U. Gühne, M. C. Angermeyer, and S. G. Riedel-Heller, "Mild cognitive impairment: Long-term course of four clinical subtypes," *Neurology* 67, no. 12 (December 2006): 2176–2185, doi: 10.1212/01.wnl.0000249117.23318.e1.

[10] "Alzheimer's disease facts and figures," Alzheimer's Association, accessed August 21, 2022, https://www.alz.org/alzheimers-dementia/facts-figures?utm_source=google&utm_medium=paidsearch&utm_campaign=google_grants&utm_content=alzheimers&gclid=Cj0KCQjw0oyYBhDGARIsAMZEuMuSo32Pcqa8dihuabni_ei5mFxUuxP-ROk6ZdPsCPNV-Nxcp-2f8qUaAlsIEALw_wcB.

[11] Jennifer J. Manly, Richard N. Jones, Kenneth M. Langa, et al., "Estimating the prevalence of dementia and mild cognitive impairment in the US: The 2016 Health and Retirement Study Harmonized Cognitive Assessment Protocol Project," *JAMA Neurology* 79, no. 12 (December 2022): 1242–1249, doi:10.1001/jamaneurol.2022.3543.

[12] Marilyn S. Albert, Steven T. DeKosky, Dennis Dickson, et al., "The diagnosis of mild cognitive impairment due to Alzheimer's disease: Recommendations from the National Institute on Aging–Alzheimer's Association workgroups on diagnostic guidelines for Alzheimer's disease," *Alzheimers & Dementia* 7, no. 3 (May 2011): 270–279, doi:10.1016/j.jalz.2011.03.008.

[13] R. C. Petersen, G. E. Smith, S. C. Waring, R. J. Ivnik, E. G. Tangalos, and E. Kokmen, "Mild cognitive impairment: Clinical characterization and outcome," *Archives of Neurology* 56, no. 3 (March 1999): 303–308, doi:10.1001/archneur.56.3.303.

"What should I do?" Sandy asked.

"I would start taking care of things. I would start getting your life in order," he replied.

Sandy was weeping when she returned to the waiting room and saw Daryl. He quickly stood up and embraced her. Sobbing, Sandy informed him that she had resolved to end her life. How, when, and under exactly what conditions remained to be determined.

Sandy—being Sandy—told her various friends and family members about the diagnosis and her intention to commit suicide before becoming completely incapacitated. She was entirely forthright with Daryl, her adult children, and other intimates. She was determined to make her wish to die "a public process, a collective experience."

Over the next year and a half, Sandy's memory and other cognitive deficits worsened to the point that a neurologist made the formal diagnosis of Alzheimer's disease. She left her position as a professor at Cornell University but continued seeing a small number of private psychotherapy patients in her home office.

*****

In November of 2010, she settled down in the living room to study two books that Daryl had dropped off. While both are basically suicide manuals, they provide the following precaution for their readers:

HELP IS AVAILABLE! If you feel that you do not fit the specified audience for our book and need emotional/psychological help, please consider the phone numbers:

USA: National Suicide Prevention Hotline USA on 1 800 273 8255, or you can call or text the National Suicide Prevention Lifeline on 988, chat on 988lifeline.org, or text HOME to 741741 to connect with a crisis counselor.

NL: 113 Suicide Prevention on 0800 0113

UK: Samaritans on 116 123, or email jo@samaritans.org or jo@samaritans.ie.

Canada: Crisis Services on 1 833 456 4566

Ireland: NOSP on 016352139

Australia: Lifeline on 13 11 14

NZ: Suicide Prevention NZ on 0508 828 865

Other international helplines can be found at befrienders.org

The first book was *Final Exit* (the most recent edition is *Final Exit 2020* and is published online), written by Derek Humphry, an English journalist whose wife developed a malignant breast cancer.[14] Humphry acquiesced to his spouse's request that he acquire a lethal dose of barbiturates from a physician-acquaintance,

---

[14] "Final Exit," Wikipedia, accessed August 21, 2022, https://en.wikipedia.org/wiki/Final_Exit.

and he was present at her side when she ingested the pills and ended her life.[15] Humphry would later emigrate to California, where, in 1980, he founded the Hemlock Society.[16]

The dual aims of the Hemlock Society were to provide information to dying people who thought about accelerating their deaths and to help pass legislation permitting carefully regulated physician-assisted dying—two different but related things. The synonyms for the latter include death with dignity (a positively valenced term favored by proponents), medical (or physician) aid in dying, physician-assisted suicide (a negatively valenced term favored by opponents), voluntary assisted dying, physician-assisted dying, and medical assistance in dying (MAiD).[17,18] Each of these is used throughout this book.

According to author Richard Côté, at its peak the Hemlock Society had 57,000 dues-paying members in 86 chapters in the United States.[19] Côté wrote, "The self-deliverance genie had been forever freed from its bottle and taken on a robust, self-sustaining life of its own."[20]

Dr. Jack Kevorkian, mainly known as "Doctor Death," but also "the euthanasia lightning rod,"[21] was a contemporary of Humphry. Dr. Kevorkian argued that "self-deliverance" was an unfortunate idea and that suffering people should ideally be offered knowledgeable aid by professionals—like himself—to peacefully, rapidly, and effectively die under supervision. This medicalized approach has been widely accepted, although in Switzerland and Austria assisted dying is currently considered a civil rather than a medical act.[22,23]

---

[15] Derek Humphry, Ann Wickett, *Jean's Way* (New York: Quartet Books, 1978).

[16] "Hemlock Society," Wikipedia, accessed August 21, 2022, https://en.wikipedia.org/wiki/Hemlock_Society.

[17] Margaret P. Battin, Thaddeus M. Pope, and Lonny Shavelson, "Medical aid in dying: Ethical and legal issues," UpToDate, accessed August 13, 2023, https://www.uptodate.com/contents/medical-aid-in-dying-ethical-and-legal-issues?search=aid%20in%20dying&source=search_result&selectedTitle=2~150&usage_type=default&display_rank=2.

[18] Thomas J. Reilly and Lauren B. Solberg. "Value of and value in language: Ethics and semantics in physician-assisted suicide laws," *The American Journal of Bioethics* 23, no. 9 (2023): 40–42.

[19] "Sudden death of writer Dick Cote," Assisted Dying Blog, accessed August 22, 2022, https://assisted-dying.org/blog/2015/02/26/sudden-death-of-writer-dick-cote/.

[20] Richard N. Cote, *In Search of Gentle Death: The Fight for Your Right to Die with Dignity* (Mt. Pleasant, SC: Corinthian Books, 2012).

[21] Associated Press, "Kevorkian a lightning rod for debate, controversy," *Charleston Gazette-Mail*, accessed August 22, 2022, https://www.wvgazettemail.com/kevorkian-a-lightning-rod-for-debate-controversy/article_4d11a5dd-f221-5024-8325-b83277fa57de.html.

[22] Preston, Nancy, Sheila Payne, and Suzanne Ost, "Breaching the stalemate on assisted dying: It's time to move beyond a medicalised approach," *British Medical Journal* 382 (2023): 1968.

[23] Claudia Gamondi, Murielle Pott, Nancy Preston, and Sheila Payne, "Family caregivers' reflections on experiences of assisted suicide in Switzerland: A qualitative interview study," *Journal of Pain and Symptom Management* 55, no. 4 (2018): 1085–1094.

On the one occasion that he met Humphry, Dr. Kevorkian invited him to refer all the Hemlock members. When the Englishman refused and stated, "I don't think we can at one and the same time be an acceptable campaigner for law reform on this issue while also blatantly breaking the law," Dr. Kevorkian became incensed and stormed out of the office.[24] Before finally being imprisoned, Dr. Kevorkian had euthanized or assisted more than 130 people to die.

The very first individual in this series was Janet Adkins, 54, from Portland, Oregon.[25,26] In 1990, her husband and two of their three sons held a press conference, and Mr. Adkins read a suicide note his wife had written several hours before her death: "I have decided for the following reasons to take my own life. This is a decision taken in a normal state of mind and is fully considered. I have Alzheimer's disease and I do not want to let it progress any further. I do not want to put my family or myself through the agony of this terrible disease."[27]

The sons did not support her decision, Mr. Adkins said. However, he fully agreed with his wife's position and accompanied her throughout the process recommended by Dr. Kevorkian, which included her initially volunteering to participate in a reputable Alzheimer's research study. It was only after the experimental trial failed that the right-to-die pioneer agreed to help hasten her death.

"They'll all be after me for this," Dr. Kevorkian said in a *New York Times* interview.[28] He described inserting an intravenous tube in Mrs. Adkins's arm and how she pressed a button that stopped the saline drip and replaced it with thiopental. This resulted in her becoming unconscious, and, after a minute, the homemade device automatically switched to a potassium chloride solution. Her heart then ceased beating.

"My ultimate aim is to make euthanasia a positive experience," the doctor explained, "I'm trying to knock the medical profession into accepting its responsibilities, and those responsibilities include assisting their patients with death."

Dr. Kevorkian and others pointed out that the word "euthanasia," derived from the Greek expression for a "good death," was debased in the America of the 1920s and Nazi Germany in the 1930s, when thousands of mentally deficient

---

[24] D. Humphry, *Good Life, Good Death: The Memoir of a Right to Die Pioneer* (New York: Carrel, 2017).

[25] Neal Nicol and Harry Wylie, *Between the Dying and the Dead: Dr. Jack Kevorkian's Life and the Battle to Legalize Euthanasia* (Co-published Columbus, Nebraska: Vision/Terrace Books, 2006).

[26] Susan Clevenger, *Dying to Die – The Janet Adkins Story: A True Story of Dying with the Assistance of Doctor Jack Kevorkian* (Maui: Sacred Life Publishers, 2019).

[27] Lisa Belkin, "Doctor tells of first death using his suicide device," *The New York Times*, accessed October 25, 2022, https://www.nytimes.com/1990/06/06/us/doctor-tells-of-first-death-using-his-suicide-device.html.

[28] Ibid.

children and adults were sterilized or put to death.[29] These acts of eugenics were then followed during World War II by the genocide of millions of Jews, non-Aryans, homosexuals, and Communists.

Although Dr. Kevorkian remains a hero to many, he was unquestionably an evangelist and a highly polarizing figure. Garnering harsh criticism for his publicity-seeking compulsion, he especially antagonized physicians and politicians. But both Dr. Kevorkian and Humphry were charismatic and eloquent individuals who launched the modern right-to-die movement in the United States and globally.[30]

In 1997, beginning with the case of *Washington v. Glucksberg*, the U.S. Supreme Court issued rulings that aid-in-dying was not something to be determined on a federal level but would require separate legalization by each of the 50 states.[31] For much of the 20th century, individual state legislatures had been debating these bills without successfully passing any of them. It became apparent to advocates that the American legislative process would require an extremely circumscribed law.

It is said that a wise politician would rather have 80% of something than 100% of nothing, or, as Barbara Coombs Lee wrote to me (January 11, 2023), "The best laws find and hold the golden center between polar political perspectives. Holding the compassionate center is the great success of medical aid in dying as conceived and implemented in Oregon some 25 years ago."

To achieve this goal the Hemlock Society activists and other proponents from Oregon arrived at four compromises. They were (1) physicians would assume the dominant role in the proposed protocol, (2) it would be limited to terminally ill patients who were going to die regardless of any treatment within the next 6 months, (3) mental capacity/competence had to be present, and (4) only oral medications were to be prescribed, and these would be ingested by self-administration.

Humphry was among the few discussants who strongly disagreed with the final concession because he also wanted people to have access to *voluntary euthanasia* (he and I discussed this together in an August 2011 interview). Euthanasia

[29] Ibid.

[30] "I never lost sight of what I wanted": An interview with right-to-die pioneer Derek Humphry," Death with Dignity, accessed September 23, 2022, https://deathwithdignity.org/news/2019/10/an-interview-with-right-to-die-pioneer-derek-humphry/.

[31] Barry F. Rosen, "Supreme Court finds no constitutional right to physician-assisted dying," Gordon Feinblatt, Attorneys at Law, January 31, 1997, accessed August 21, 2022, https://www.gfrlaw.com/what-we-do/insights/supreme-court-finds-no-constitutional-right-physician-assisted-dying#:~:text=Health%20Law%20TOPICS-,Supreme%20Court%20Finds%20No%20Constitutional%20Right%20to%20Physician%2DAssisted%20Dying,a%20physician's%20assistance%20to%20die.

entails the administration—most often intravenously—of lethal drugs by medical practitioners at the request of a suffering individual, and this approach is currently legal in Canada, Belgium, Luxembourg, and the Netherlands. By contrast, self-ingestion of oral medications is the method employed in Austria, Germany, Italy, New Zealand, Portugal, Spain, and Australia.[32] Data from Canada find that when patients are given a choice between either voluntary euthanasia or self-ingestion, the overwhelming majority chose the former.

The explanation for this last finding is not simple.

Canadian activist Dr. Chantal Perrot remarked to me (September 2, 2022): "That is partly because [euthanasia] is all most of us offer. There are oral protocols, but they are more time-consuming and less predictable, and there are different regulations in each province and territory regarding clinician supervision/presence for the oral ingestion. [Furthermore], the oral meds are not paid for in all regions, whereas the IV meds are."

But, I would add, it also makes psychological sense to me that most people would request intravenous administration by a knowledgeable and kindly authority figure (i.e., a doctor or nurse practitioner) rather than ingest a lethal dose of medications by themselves. Gallup's annual Values and Beliefs poll has consistently found in recent years that Americans broadly support euthanasia, which they measure by inquiring, "When a person has a disease that cannot be cured, do you think doctors should be allowed by law to end the patient's life by some painless means if the patient and his or her family request it?" In 2020, this was endorsed by 71% of respondents, while the physician-assisted dying question was affirmed by 61% of the sample who agreed that "doctors should be allowed to assist such patients in committing suicide if they request it."[33]

However, as the Oregon bill was being formulated, some advocates argued that the word "euthanasia"—whether the act was voluntary or not—is irreparably tainted and would likely scuttle the ballot measure. Consequently, this method was dropped from the draft of the bill. The resulting Oregon Death with Dignity Act became a citizen's initiative that narrowly passed in November of 1994 with 51% of voter endorsement. Implementation was delayed by legal proceedings, but in the next ballot initiative 60% of the electorate reaffirmed the Act, which was finally implemented in 1997.[34]

[32] Sean Riley, "Watching the watchmen: Changing tides in the oversight of medical assistance in dying," *Journal of Medical Ethics* 49, no. 7 (2023): 453–457.

[33] Jeffrey M. Jones, "Prevalence of living wills in U.S. up slightly," *Gallup*, accessed October 5, 2023, https://news.gallup.com/poll/312209/prevalence-living-wills-slightly.aspx.

[34] "Death with Dignity Act," Oregon Health Authority, accessed August 25, 2022, https://www.oregon.gov/oha/ph/providerpartnerresources/evaluationresearch/deathwithdignityact/pages/index.aspx.

Of direct relevance to Dan, the Oregon criteria was tailored especially for people dying from cancer, *and it excluded most people with dementing illnesses or other neurodegenerative disorders and related chronic conditions.* All subsequent American death-with-dignity laws—and there are a total of 10 states and the District of Columbia that have currently legalized the practice—are based on the original Oregon legislation. Cultural anthropologist Anita Hannig is not alone in her unfortunate but somewhat exaggerated assessment "that America has the strictest assisted dying laws in the world. . . . The letter of the law continues to stifle patients who are either too sick or not sick enough to qualify for a prescription."[35]

The second book Sandy perused was *The Peaceful Pill Handbook*, written by the visionary Australian physician Philip Nitschke and his partner, Fiona Stewart.[36] The authors discussed how doctors therapeutically prescribed barbiturates as sleeping pills, but the potential for dependency issues and accidental deaths eventually led clinicians to abandon this practice. However, Dr. Nitschke and Stewart wrote that one could still obtain and employ Nembutal, a brand name for pentobarbital, as a means to end one's life. This is a liquid barbiturate used by veterinarians to euthanize animals, and there was an active black market for the drug. When Sandy was dealing with her Alzheimer's, people were primarily recommending Mexican sources to acquire Nembutal, and couriers either transported the drug over the border from Tijuana or covertly used the U.S. Postal Service after ordering it online. The diminutive psychologist successfully obtained Nembutal by means of the latter approach, but it is important to understand that, at present, this route has mainly been taken over by scam artists from China and other countries. It is no longer recommended by Nitschke, Stewart, and others.[37]

*****

Karen, Sandy's neighbor, came up with the idea of gathering the Bems' inner circle of friends on the Sunday before she intended to die. A small group assembled in the diminutive psychotherapist's living room and plunked down on couches to talk about her life. Humorous "Sandy stories" were recounted while she listened intently. According to Karen, Daryl was always an accomplished

[35] Anita Hannig, *The Day I Die: The Untold Story of Assisted Dying in America* (Naperville, IL: Sourcebooks, 2022).

[36] Philip Nitschke and Fiona Stewart, "The Peaceful Pill Handbook – Essentials Edition," The Peaceful Pill Handbook, accessed August 25, 2022, https://www.peacefulpillhandbook.com/about-the-handbook/.

[37] Colin Brewer, *Let Me Not Get Alzheimer's, Sweet Heaven!* (Waswichshire, UK: Skyscraper Publications, 2019).

raconteur, and he enthralled the group with anecdotes about how his wife had brashly testified in key court cases. He colorfully described her numerous professional successes, and her loving efforts on behalf of their children. Karen and the others took turns reminiscing, and Sandy would frequently interject to ask, "Wow, I did that? Amazing! Amazing!" At other points, she would smile broadly and exclaim, "Wait! I *really* did *that*?"

There was much laughter and weeping in the room. Sandy was the center of attention, surrounded by those who loved her. Throughout the evening, she vacillated between being incredulous and ecstatic.

Two days later, Sandy sat down at her desk and reviewed a brief document she had printed. It explicitly stated why and how she was going to die. She then got out a pen and wrote the date, May 20, 2014, followed by the words: "The time has come to end my life. I love you, Daryl." She then signed the bottom of the page.

Later, her husband watched while she used a pair of manicure scissors to carefully open the package containing Nembutal, which had successfully arrived. Pouring the contents into a goblet, she placed it on her nightstand alongside a glass of wine.

Climbing into bed, Sandy confusedly gazed at the two glasses. "Which," she asked Daryl, "is the drug? Which is the wine?"

"The drug is clear, and the wine is red," he explained.

Forgetting his response, Sandy repeated the question. After he patiently answered again, Sandy then inquired whether she could sip some of the drug and then drink some of the wine. He told her that it would *not* be a good idea because she might fall asleep before entirely finishing the medication. At that point, she promptly drank down all the barbiturate and the full glass of wine.

Daryl told me: "She asked if I would get into the bed with her . . . I held her and could hear her breathing. I just sort of watched every moment . . . until her breathing stopped."

Sandy's obituary in the *Pittsburgh-Post Gazette* was honest and in-your-face, like the woman herself.[38] It explicitly stated that she had committed suicide with pentobarbital after having been diagnosed with Alzheimer's disease 4 years earlier.

During her memorial service, Daryl would later recite from Fred Chappell's poem, "Difference," the following lines: "The armchair seems not empty but

---

[38] "Obituary: Sandra Bem/Psychologist, feminist, pioneer in gender roles," *Pittsburgh Post-Gazette*, accessed May 23, 2014, https://www.post-gazette.com/news/obituaries/2014/05/23/Obituary-Sandra-Bem-Psychologist-feminist-pioneer-in-gender-roles/stories/201405230080.

incomplete / And the patch of sunlit rug unoccupied / More vacant than the sky when the moon is hid / In the cavern of December's longest night."[39]

As I considered these events, I thought: *Most people with Alzheimer's disease die twice. First their identity dissolves—higher-order thinking is gone although the brainstem continues to operate and sustain heart and lungs. Only later their body deteriorates, and the vital organs finally cease functioning.*[40,41]

Sally Thorne, RN, PhD, a professor from the School of Nursing and Principal Research Chair in Palliative and End-of-Life Care at the University of British Columbia (interview July 5, 2023) captured this distinction by explaining that there is no agreed upon definition of death in modern healthcare, leaving us in a conceptual transition between death as a primarily biological event and death as a primarily social event. "Nurses are especially interested in understanding how meaningful life and personhood fade away during social deaths," she told me, "and how this contributes to the suffering of families and the individual."

Dan said that after reading *The New York Times Magazine* article, he only wished he could tell Sandy Bem, "Thank you."

Dan explained, "It was a mesmerizing story. . . . I hadn't been walking around with the certainty I was going to become an Alzheimer's patient, but I just assumed it. I read about Sandy shortly after my dad died and couldn't tear my eyes from the pages. Her voice was my voice. She did what I wanted to do. The support she had from her husband was the support I needed to receive."

He considered her to be his "role model." He admired Sandy Bem for many things, but especially because she was forthright with her loved ones. Dan read and reread the magazine piece a dozen times. He made 20 copies to distribute to his inner circle of intimates so that they would understand what he intended to do.

It wasn't difficult for me to imagine him handing out the article.

[39] Fred Davis Chappell, "Difference," All Poetry, accessed August 26, 2022, https://allpoetry.com/poem/15087097-Difference-by-Fred-Davis-Chappell.

[40] Ryan Montoya, "What is death, exactly?," *Scientific America*, accessed July 4, 2023, https://blogs.scientificamerican.com/observations/what-is-death-exactly/.

[41] Barbara Pesut and Sally Thorne, "Reflections on the relational ontology of medical assistance in dying," *Nursing Philosophy* e12438 (April 2023), https://doi.org/10.1111/nup.12438.

8

Dan and John were incredibly compatible, and they both soothed and healed each other. The two men had independently learned the same life lesson: the only way you can possibly reach people is with an open, honest heart. This understanding had given each of them another shot at love. It gave them a common foundation from which to tackle their challenges together. It would allow John to continue emerging from a profound depression and Dan to confront the resurgence of his earlier traumas while continuing efforts at reconciling with his nuclear family.

Over a 10-year period, the two men formed a productive partnership. They decided to sell Dan's first condominium in the city. Tapping into John's architectural design skills, the couple built themselves a new house in the Laurelhurst neighborhood. Later, anticipating how dementia would continue to impact Dan's ability to function independently, they sold the house and moved to the more vibrant community of Chinatown. John also rented a studio near the apartment and began producing a series of attractive monochromatic ink drawings, one of which forms the basis of this book's cover illustration.

"Because of the AIDS epidemic, death has been too much of a factor in John's life," Dan would wryly tell me. "I'm just gob-smacked by the kind of support he gives me. It's nothing short of heroic." John felt exactly the same way about Dan.

*****

Dan always assumed that one day he would be diagnosed with Alzheimer's, but he had deferred pursuing a neurological evaluation. In a study conducted by the Alzheimer's Society of the United Kingdom, more than half (56%) of people similarly put off seeking a dementia diagnosis for up to a year or more. The explanation for this behavior is likely linked to two other findings in the research: almost two-thirds of people surveyed (62%) felt that the diagnosis would mean their life was over, and dementia is the most feared health condition after cancer in the United States and the United Kingdom.[1–3]

According to Rabbi Jonathan Romain, the director of the Maidenhead Synagogue in Berkshire, England: "When I first became a rabbi, the main fear everyone had was developing cancer. But we have learned to live with that. Now what terrifies congregants most is Alzheimer's, which can not only destroy a once-intelligent person but shatter their relationship with partners or children."[4]

Dan's good friend, Drew, told me he always considered the man from Kansas to be "an absent-minded guy, who was not especially adept with computers or cellphones." But Dan's forgetfulness was considerably more evident in 2015, when he joined Drew and Pauline on an African safari. John did not accompany them, but he, too, had been noticing that his husband's memory was slipping.

However, it was Dan's older son who was most concerned. In late 2017, he urged Dan to see a neuropsychologist, explaining, "You're repeating yourself. You're forgetting things that we've just planned. You're forgetting basic things. You're forgetting things across the board."

Dan told me, "I was also having trouble reading, so I listened to his advice." In December, a general practitioner made him an appointment with a Portland neuropsychologist to undergo testing.

According to Dr. Booker Bush, a primary care physician from Baystate Medical Center in Springfield, Massachusetts (email January 31, 2023), "I think the biggest mistake you can make in medicine is arriving at a difficult diagnosis by yourself. It's frequently useful to have a sub-specialist either broaden your diagnostic possibilities or confirm your diagnostic impressions.[5] Neuropsychologists have expertise in differentiating whether somebody is having problems with memory concentration and focus because of 'hardwiring' of the brain, e.g., strokes and neurodegenerative disorders, or due to brain 'software,' e.g., major depression, ADHD, emotional trauma, etc."

---

[1] "What medical condition are you most afraid of?," Medicare Advantage, accessed April 17, 2023, https://www.medicareadvantage.com/news/most-feared-heath-conditions-report#:~:text= The%20Top%205%20Most%20Feared,%2C%20strokes%20and%20COVID%2D19.&text=Can cer%20fears%20are%20more%20than%20justified.

[2] "Over half of people fear dementia diagnosis, 62 per cent think it means 'life is over,'" Alzheimer's Society, accessed October 8, 2022, https://www.alzheimers.org.uk/news/2018-05-29/over-half-people-fear-dementia-diagnosis-62-cent-think-it-means-life-over.

[3] Dan G. Blazer, Krstine Yaffe, and Jason Karlawish, "Cognitive aging: A report from the Institute of Medicine," *JAMA* 313, no. 21 (June 2015): 2121–2122, doi: 10.1001/jama.2015.4380.

[4] JC Reporter, "'It's just like looking after a toddler': Dementia carers share their experiences," Jewish Chronicle, June 9, 2023, https://www.thejc.com/news/community/its-just-like-looking-after-a-toddler-dementia-carers-share-their-experiences-5GsNNdDCH8VDpDMFESoPkp.

[5] Robin Levinson-King, "'There was no hope': Treatable disease often mistaken for Alzheimer's," *BBC News*, accessed March 25, 2023, https://www.bbc.com/news/world-us-canada-49375308.

After taking a 2-day battery of exams, Dan explained, "I was completely convinced that I had aced them."

He hadn't.

The 57-year-old man was informed that, like Sandy Bem, he had a significant Mild Cognitive Impairment (MCI). Dan had become one of the roughly 2 million Americans with the diagnosis.

Later, brain imaging purportedly revealed the presence of amyloid plaques, and a neurologist would point them out and declare, "Those tiny dark grains of sand in your brain? That's the Alzheimer's." During the subsequent consultation, Dan officially took his place among the roughly 6 million Americans who have received the diagnosis of full-fledged Alzheimer's dementia.[6]

Incidentally, I don't understand what was meant by the reference to "grains of sand," as plaques are mostly a pathological finding at autopsy and not something that's evident on *ordinary* radiological scans. It is possible—but not probable—according to Dr. Zachary Macchi (November 2, 2022, interview), a neurologist from the University of Colorado, that the "grains" were microhemorrhages suggestive of cerebral amyloid angiopathy. But in any case, Alzheimer's is a clinical-pathologic diagnosis based on history and impaired functioning, and it is generally confirmed postmortem—that is after one's death—by a histopathological examination of the brain cells.

However, according to Dr. Georges Naasan (October 27, 2022, interview), Medical Director for the division of Behavioral Neurology and Neuropsychiatry at Mount Sinai Hospital in New York, "We live in a day and age where we can confirm with a hundred percent certainty whether someone has Alzheimer's disease, and this can be done through a spinal tap or a special PET scan image."[7,8] Dr. Naasan told me that the first approach takes advantage of biomarkers. After inserting a needle into the back, fluid is removed "and sent to the lab where it's examined for the proteins associated with Alzheimer's disease—mainly beta-amyloid 42 (the major component of amyloid plaques in the brain), tau, and phospho-tau. Through an examination of the levels of the protein in the cerebrospinal fluid, we can determine with, like, a 99% accuracy, I won't say a hundred,

[6] "Alzheimer's disease facts and figures," Alzheimer's Association, accessed December 7, 2022, https://www.alz.org/alzheimers-dementia/facts-figures?utm_source=google&utm_medium=paidsearch&utm_campaign=google_grants&utm_content=alzheimers&gclid=EAIaIQobChMIidxyvHn-wIVj4vICh0wlg84EAAYASAAEgJTbPD_BwE.

[7] Victor L. Villemagne, Vincent Doré, Samantha Burnham, Colin L. Masters, and Christopher Rowe, "Imaging tau and amyloid-beta proteinopathies in Alzheimer disease and other conditions," *Nature Reviews Neurology* 14, no. 4 (April 2018): 225–236, doi: 10.1038/nrneurol.2018.9.

[8] Willemijn J. Jansen, Olin Janssen, Betty Tijms, et al., "Prevalence estimates of amyloid abnormality across the Alzheimer disease clinical spectrum," *JAMA Neurology* 79, no. 3 (March 2022): 228–243, doi: 10.1001/jamaneurol.2021.5216.

you know, that was a little bit of a stretch, but 99% accuracy, whether that person has Alzheimer's disease or doesn't."[9]

"The second modality," he continued, "involves an unusual type of imaging called an amyloid PET scan. Instead of taking fluid out and measuring the level of the proteins, we inject patients with a material that has two properties. The first is an affinity to amyloid that allows it to latch onto a plaque, if present, in your brain. The second property is that it's radioactive and will light up on the image."

"How commonly are these performed?" I asked.

Dr. Naasan responded that while they may be regularly used in research investigations or when the clinical picture is unusual, they are otherwise rarely employed.

"Why?"

"The spinal tap involves inserting a large-bore needle in your back between two of your bones, which is uncomfortable and carries risks." He went on to say, "And because the amyloid PET scan isn't covered by any insurance and costs about $5,000, there are not a lot of people who can or want to afford such an expensive procedure."

It is highly unlikely Dan underwent either of these, and I suspect that his diagnosis was determined on the basis of neuropsychological testing, medical history, and physical examination. He had at least one of the dementias, but I am uncertain as to whether he solely met the criteria for Alzheimer's disease.

According to Diana Waugh, RN: "We call a lot of memory loss 'Alzheimer's', and I'll tell you why! First, for a long time there was no other billing code. If a physician saw your loved one and there were memory problems, they tagged it Alzheimer's, so they could get paid. . . . I'm not being negative about physicians . . . I understand they need to be paid. [But] we've gotten kind of a skewed view that it's all Alzheimer's. I don't really much care, to be totally honest."[10,11]

However, we should care, because diagnostic clarity is necessary if we are ever going to be able to identify the trajectories or discover cures for the different types of dementing illnesses.

*****

[9] "How biomarkers help diagnose dementia," National Institute on Aging, accessed December 7, 2022, https://www.nia.nih.gov/health/how-biomarkers-help-diagnose-dementia.

[10] Diana Waugh, "How to talk to someone with dementia," mmlearn.org, accessed November 15, 2022, https://www.youtube.com/watch?v=ilickabmjww.

[11] Diana Waugh, *I Was Thinking: Unlocking the Door to Successful Conversations with Loved Ones with Cognitive Loss* (Lulu.com, 2008).

After meeting with the neurologist, Dan sat down with John for a serious conversation. Because of Dan's experience with his father's illness, he had no intention of slowly dying from progressive dementia. Instead, like Sandy Bem, he intended to inform the rest of his family and closest friends that he would be preparing a plan to end his life. Like Sandy, he was going to overdose with medications.

In our very first interview, Dan calmly declared, "I'm going take my own life before I am unable. You've got to give up good time to be able to succeed. You have to end your life when you have the capacity to do it yourself. . . . I'm trying to decide when that time is."

"So, what will be the marker for you?" I asked.

"The key," he said, "is hitting that note, hitting that date. If only there is some way to figure out after which day I'm not going to be cognitively capable of doing this. If November 15th is that date, I will do it on the 14th."

Dan hadn't fully answered my question, and probably he couldn't.

The reporter Stephen P. Kiernan has observed: "Dozens of people taught me that same lesson during my research. They did not fear death, but they feared dying badly. They did not want to live forever, but they wanted to live well for as long as possible. They did not want to die one moment too soon, but they did not want to suffer one moment too long."[12]

Kiernan and Dan were touching on a phenomenon that some people in the right-to-die community have begun to call "Five minutes to midnight," while others have labeled "Ten minutes to midnight."[13,14] In either case, the phrase is borrowed from the story of Cinderella, and it refers to our understandable urge to hang on until the last moment at the Grand Ball before the clock strikes 12, the ornate carriage turns into a pumpkin, the horses into mice, and our elegant gown reverts back into rags.

*****

After he received the diagnosis, Dan went looking to see if the medical treatment of Alzheimer's had improved since his father's time.

It hadn't.

He learned from a newly published study that, worldwide, there are 57 million people living with dementia, and the number is going to explode over the

[12] Stephen P. Kiernan, *Last Rights: Rescuing the End of Life from the Medical System* (New York: St. Martin's Press, 2006), 275.

[13] Andrew Bomford and Estelle Doyle, "Wanting to die at 'five to midnight': Before dementia takes over," *BBC News*, accessed September 22, 2022, https://www.bbc.com/news/stories-47047579.

[14] "B.C. man is one of the first Canadians with dementia to die with medical assistance," CBC Radio, accessed September 23, 2022, https://www.cbc.ca/radio/sunday/the-sunday-edition-for-october-27-2019-1.5335017/b-c-man-is-one-of-the-first-canadians-with-dementia-to-die-with-medical-assistance-1.5335025.

next couple of decades as the Earth's population continues to age.[15] Japan, which has the highest proportion of people 65 or older in the world, is leading a global demographic trend. However, an average of 10,000 American boomers are turning 65 each day, and by the year 2034 there will be more older Americans than children.[16-18] Around 1 in 4 people who are currently 55 years and older have a close birth relative with dementia,[19] and 1 in 10 Americans over 65 are diagnosed with this clinical condition.[20] "Dementia" is a general term for loss of memory. "Neurodegenerative disease" is an umbrella term that includes the dementias, but also such disorders as Lou Gehrig's disease (amyotrophic lateral sclerosis) and Parkinson's disease.[21]

According to Alfonso Fasano, MD (November 4, 2022, interview), a neurologist from the University of Toronto, all these conditions are caused by progressive damage to cells and nervous system connections that are necessary for cognition, mobility, coordination, and other different brain functions. There are dozens of disorders with different etiologies that result in dementia, of which Alzheimer's disease accounts for 60–70% of cases.[22] Others include vascular dementia, Down syndrome, frontotemporal dementia,[23] Wernicke-Korsakoff

[15] Emma Nichols, Jaimie D. Steinmetz, Stein Emil Vollset, et al., "Estimation of the global prevalence of dementia in 2019 and forecasted prevalence in 2050: An analysis for the Global Burden of Disease Study 2019," *Lancet* 7, no. 2 (January 2022): E105–E124, https://doi.org/10.1016/S2468-2667(21)00249-8.

[16] The Editorial Board, "Can America age gracefully?," *The New York Times*, accessed September 1, 2023, https://www.nytimes.com/interactive/2023/09/06/opinion/seniors-old-age-america.html.

[17] J. R. Knickman and E. K. Snell. "The 2030 problem: Caring for aging baby boomers," *Health Services Research* 37, no. 4 (August 2002): 848–884, doi: 10.1034/j.1600-0560.2002.56.x. PMID: 12236388; PMCID: PMC1464018.

[18] "Baby boomer," Wikipedia, accessed October 29, 2022, https://en.wikipedia.org/wiki/Baby_boomers.

[19] "Can genes cause dementia?," Alzheimer's Association, accessed June 21, 2023, https://www.alzheimers.org.uk/about-dementia/risk-factors-and-prevention/can-genes-cause-dementia.

[20] Jennifer J. Manly, Richard N. Jones, Kenneth M. Langa, et al., "Estimating the prevalence of dementia and mild cognitive impairment in the US: The 2016 Health and Retirement Study Harmonized Cognitive Assessment Protocol Project," *JAMA Neurology* 79, no. 12 (December 2022): 1242–1249, doi: 10.1001/jamaneurol.2022.3543.

[21] Yujun Hou, Xiuli Dan, Mansi Babbar, et al., "Ageing as a risk factor for neurodegenerative disease," *Nature Reviews Neurology* 15, no. 10 (October 2019): 565–581, https://doi.org/10.1038/s41582-019-0244-7.

[22] "Dementia," World Health Organization, accessed September 22, 2022, https://www.who.int/news-room/fact-sheets/detail/dementia.

[23] "Providing care for a person with a frontotemporal disorder," National Institute on Aging, accessed October 24, 2022, https://www.nia.nih.gov/health/providing-care-person-frontotemporal-disorder.

syndrome resulting from vitamin B$_1$ deficiency associated with alcoholism,[24] Huntington's disease,[25] and the Lewy body dementias.[26–28]

Chronic traumatic encephalopathy (CTE) has recently received considerable publicity. The condition is associated with repeated blows to the head during combat or when athletes engage in contact sports (i.e., football, rugby, boxing, soccer, etc.). Research breakthroughs are speeding up the development of an identifying test for this type of dementia.[29]

Otherwise, in much the same way that the words "cancer" and "AIDS" were barely mentioned 30 years ago, the diagnosis of dementia has also been similarly stigmatized.[30] Given the enormous prevalence of dementia, only a relatively small number of public figures have been identified as having Alzheimer's disease: President Ronald Reagan, former first lady Rosalynn Carter, Prime Minister Margaret Thatcher, the singer Glen Campbell, the author Terry Pratchett, and the basketball coach Pat Summitt. In addition, the actors Joanne Woodward and Gene Wilder come to mind. Before Tony Bennett's death in 2023, his family acknowledged that he was suffering from the disease, and his wife, Susan, announced, "He's not the old Tony anymore. But when he sings, he's the old Tony."[31] Both Robin Williams's dementia with Lewy bodies and Bruce Willis's frontotemporal dementia have also received a fair amount of

---

[24] "Wernicke-Korsakoff syndrome," National Institute of Neurological Disorders and Stroke, accessed November 27, 2022, https://www.ninds.nih.gov/health-information/disorders/wernicke-korsakoff-syndrome#:~:text=Korsakoff%20syndrome%20(also%20called%20Korsakoff's,the%20brain%20involved%20with%20memory.

[25] Jennie Erin Smith, "Sought out by science, and then forgotten," The New York Times, May 23, 2023, https://www.nytimes.com/2023/05/23/science/huntingtons-disease-colombia.html?campaign_id=34&emc=edit_sc_20230523&instance_id=93214&nl=science-times&regi_id=63340269&segment_id=133678&te=1&user_id=895343099129dcd1f95fa65a5a136796.

[26] "Research Centers of Excellence," LBDA, accessed October 24, 2022, https://www.lbda.org/research/research-centers-of-excellence/#.

[27] "Lewy body dementias," Wikipedia, accessed September 23, 2022, https://en.wikipedia.org/wiki/Lewy_body_dementias.

[28] D. Avramopoulos, D. Kapogiannis, J. M. Leoutsakos, et al., "Developing treatments for Alzheimer's and related disorders with precision medicine: A vision," Advances in Experimental Medicine and Biology 1339 (January 2021): 395–402, doi: 10.1007/978-3-030-78787-5_49. PMID: 35023131; PMCID: PMC9358929.

[29] Ken Belson, "A test for C.T.E. in the living may be closer than ever," The New York Times, accessed November 18, 2022, https://www.nytimes.com/2022/11/17/sports/football/cte-test-concussions-alzheimers.html.

[30] Diana Waugh, "How to talk to someone with dementia," mmlearn.org, accessed November 15, 2022, https://www.youtube.com/watch?v=ilickabmjww.

[31] Christi Carras, "Tony Bennett's family says he has Alzheimer's: 'But when he sings, he's the old Tony,'" Yahoo, accessed October 16, 2022, https://news.yahoo.com/tony-bennetts-family-says-alz heimers-165310095.html?guccounter=1.

attention, chiefly because their families want to promote awareness and encourage research.[32]

While millions of Americans carry a diagnosis of Alzheimer's disease, only 200,000 people, or 1–2%, have what is called "early-onset" Alzheimer's, which begins when they are younger than 65.[33] Alzheimer's disease is the most common type of early-onset dementia. Younger people are much more likely to have an "atypical" type of Alzheimer's disease, and their primary problems may include difficulty understanding visual information or language.[34] There is a familial type of Alzheimer's that can manifest as early as the third decade with a variety of noncognitive neurological signs and symptoms, but it is very rare.[35,36]

Dan is among the subgroup of patients with early-onset dementia, which columnist Jane E. Brody wrote is "especially traumatic and challenging for families to acknowledge, and many practicing physicians fail to suspect it may be an underlying cause of symptoms."[37] People with early-onset dementia also have special difficulty accessing appropriate healthcare as many services are tailored toward the elderly with very different medical and social needs.[38]

A family history is not necessary for an individual to develop Alzheimer's; however, research indicates that people (like Dan) who have a parent or sibling with the disorder are more likely to develop a disease than are those who do not have a first-degree relative with Alzheimer's. There are some genetic risk factors for early-onset Alzheimer's disease, including the presence of the genes

[32] Kristen Rogers, "What Robin Williams' widow wants you to know about the future of Lewy body dementia," *CNN*, accessed August 20, 2022, https://www.cnn.com/2022/07/01/health/lewy-body-dementia-robin-williams-life-itself-wellness/index.html.

[33] "Minorities and women are at greater risk for Alzheimer's disease," Centers for Disease Control and Prevention, accessed September 23, 2022, https://www.cdc.gov/aging/publications/features/Alz-Greater-Risk.html#:~:text=Current%20estimates%20are%20that%20about,65%20with%20younger%2Donset%20Alzheimer's.

[34] "What causes young-onset dementia?," Alzheimer's Association, accessed June 23, 2023, https://www.alzheimers.org.uk/about-dementia/types-dementia/what-causes-young-onset-dementia#:~:text=Alzheimer's%20disease%20is%20the%20most,plaques'%20and%20'tangles'.

[35] Liyong Wu, Pedro Rosa-Neto, Ging-Yuek R. Hsiung, et al., "Early-onset familial Alzheimer's disease (EOFAD)," *Canadian Journal of Neurological Sciences* 39, no. 4 (July 2012): 436–445, doi: 10.1017/S0317167100013949.

[36] Jesús Andrade-Guerrero, Alberto Santiago-Balmaseda, Paola Jeronimo-Aguilar, et al., "Alzheimer's disease: An updated overview of its genetics," *International Journal of Molecular Sciences* 24, no. 4 (February 2023): 3754, https://doi.org/10.3390/ijms24043754.

[37] Jane E. Brody, "When dementia strikes at an early age," *The New York Times*, accessed September 23, 2022, https://www.nytimes.com/2022/01/17/well/mind/dementia-alzheimers-younger-adults.html.

[38] Mibenge Nsenduluka, "Younger onset dementia on the rise," *Illawarra Mercury*, accessed July 28, 2022, https://www.illawarramercury.com.au/story/7837407/younger-onset-dementia-on-the-rise/.

presenillin 1, presenillin 2, and APOE4 heterozygosity.[39,40] Down syndrome is another related genetic condition, and it conveys an increased risk due to the presence of an extra allele of chromosome 21 that results in the production of an amyloid precursor protein.[41] However, nearly all cases of dementia are the result of a complex interplay between genetics and environmental and behavioral factors; genes may increase the risk of developing a dementia, but they rarely cause it directly.[42]

In a nationwide, population-based, cohort study conducted in Denmark, early-, middle-, and late-life depressive symptoms have been associated with subsequent dementia diagnoses and may be an early symptom or response to preclinical disease; however, a link between suicide risk and a dementia is unclear.[43-45] Research has reported that the subgroup of patients younger than 65 years (like Dan) is nearly three times more likely than patients without dementia to commit suicide after adjusting for age and sex.[46]

Studies have consistently found that women are disproportionately affected by Alzheimer's disease, and approximately two-thirds of all patients are female.[47]

[39] Bart De Strooper, Takeshi Iwatsubo, and Michael S. Wolfe, "Presenilins and γ-secretase: Structure, function, and role in Alzheimer disease," *Cold Spring Harbor Perspectives on Medicine* 2, no. 1 (January 2012):a006304, doi: 10.1101/cshperspect.a006304. PMID: 22315713; PMCID: PMC3253024.

[40] Robert D. Moir, Richard Lathe, and Rudolph E. Tanzi, "The antimicrobial protection hypothesis of Alzheimer's disease," *Alzheimer's & Dementia* 14, no. 12 (December 2018): 1602–1614, doi: 10.1016/j.jalz.2018.06.3040. PMID 30314800.

[41] "Alzheimer's disease in people with Down syndrome," National Institute on Aging, accessed June 14, 2023, https://www.nia.nih.gov/health/alzheimers-disease-people-down-syndrome#:~:text=Estimates%20suggest%20that%2050%25%20or,a%20parent%20to%20a%20child.

[42] "Is Alzheimer's genetic?," Alzheimer's Association, accessed June 22, 2023, https://www.alz.org/alzheimers-dementia/what-is-alzheimers/causes-and-risk-factors/genetics#:~:text=Is%20Alzheimer's%20Genetic%3F,first%2Ddegree%20relative%20with%20Alzheimer's.

[43] Holly Elser, Erzsébet Horváth-Puhó, Jaimie L. Gradus, et al., "Association of early-, middle-, and late-life depression with incident dementia in a Danish cohort," *JAMA Neurology*, published online July 24, 2023, doi: 10.1001/jamaneurol.2023.2309

[44] Annette Erlangsen, Steven H. Zarit, and Yeates Conwell, "Hospital-diagnosed dementia and suicide: A longitudinal study using prospective, nationwide register data," *American Journal of Geriatric Psychiatry* 16, no. 3 (March 2008): 220–228, doi: 10.1097/01.JGP.0000302930.75387.7e

[45] Annette Erlangsen, Egon Stenager, Yeates Conwell, et al., "Association between neurological disorders and death by suicide in Denmark," *JAMA* 323, no. 5 (February 2020): 444–454, doi: 10.1001/jama.2019.21834.

[46] Danah Alothman, Timothy Card, Sarah Lewis, et al., "Risk of suicide after dementia diagnosis," *JAMA Neurology* 79, no. 11 (October 2022): 1148–1154, https://jamanetwork.com/journals/jamaneurology/article-abstract/2796654, doi: 10.1001/jamaneurol.2022.3094.

[47] Lisa L. Barnes, Robert S. Wilson, Julia L. Bienias, et al., "Sex differences in the clinical manifestations of Alzheimer disease pathology," *Archives of General Psychiatry* 62, no. 6 (June 2005): 685–691, doi: 10.1001/archpsyc.62.6.685.

Why? On average, women live longer than men[48]; in addition, genes that contribute to the production of amyloid and tau proteins, or apolipoprotein E4 (which affects cholesterol transport within the brain), appear to have a stronger effect on women than upon men.[49,50]

Dan was described by John as being "a really white guy," and race plays a complicated role in the dementias. Investigations have consistently found that, for the overall U.S. population, Black Americans are roughly 1.5–2 times more likely than whites to develop Alzheimer's and other dementias.[51] While Hispanic older adults are less well studied, they also have a greater incidence of dementia than do white older adults.[52] However, there are several confounding variables, and Black participants in Alzheimer's disease research studies are scattered throughout the country as part of the National Institute of Aging's network of Alzheimer's Disease Research Centers. They are 35% less likely to have been diagnosed when seen at the initial intake visit than are white participants,[53] quality of medical care, referral bias, and differences in diagnostic thresholds applied by providers may each explain why national data collected over a 15-year period suggest that Black participants with Alzheimer's and related dementias have greater cognitive impairment and symptom severity than white subjects.[54]

[48] E. J. Davis, L. Broestl, S. Abdulai-Saiku, et al., "A second X chromosome contributes to resilience in a mouse model of Alzheimer's disease," *Science of Translational Medicine* 12, no. 558 (August 2020): eaaz5677, doi: 10.1126/scitranslmed.aaz5677. PMID: 32848093; PMCID: PMC8409261.

[49] Erin Reed-Geaghan, "Why does Alzheimer's disease affect more women than men?," BrightFocus Foundation, accessed January 30, 2023, https://www.brightfocus.org/alzheimers/article/why-does-alzheimers-disease-affect-more-women-men#:~:text=Women%20are%20disproportionately%20affected%20by,men%20following%20an%20AD%20diagnosis.

[50] Andrea Sturchio, et al., "High soluble amyloid-β 42 predicts normal cognition in amyloid-positive individuals with Alzheimer's disease-causing mutations," *Alzheimers Disease* 90, no. 1 (January 2022): 333–348, doi: 10.3233/JAD-220808.

[51] Jennifer Weuve, Lisa L. Barnes, Carlos F. Mendes de Leon, et al., "Cognitive aging in black and white Americans: Cognition, cognitive decline, and incidence of Alzheimer disease dementia," *Epidemiology* 29, no. 1 (January 2018): 151–159, doi: 10.1097/EDE.0000000000000747. PMID: 28863046; PMCID: PMC5718953.

[52] Erica Kornblith, Amber Bahorik, W. John Boscardin, et al., "Association of race and ethnicity with incidence of dementia among older adults," *JAMA* 327, no. 15 (April 2022): 1488–1495, doi: 10.1001/jama.2022.3550.

[53] "Data shows racial disparities in Alzheimer's disease diagnosis between Black and white research study participants," National Institute of Aging, accessed January 31, 2023, https://www.nia.nih.gov/news/data-shows-racial-disparities-alzheimers-disease-diagnosis-between-black-and-white-research.

[54] Jack C. Lennon, Stephen L. Aita, Victor A. Del Bene, et al., "Black and white individuals differ in dementia prevalence, risk factors, and symptomatic presentation," *Alzheimer's & Dementia* 18, no. 8 (August 2022): 1461–1471, https://doi.org/10.1002/alz.12509.

The "amyloid hypothesis" is the most widely discussed paradigm for the eti-ology of Alzheimer's disease.[55,56] Mainly based on autopsy and genetic data, the hypothesis postulates that misprocessing of amyloid precursor protein leads to the creation of toxic peptides. These assemble into oligomers and deposit into plaques, which result in synaptic degeneration and the emergence of tau phos-phorylation within neurons. The death of neurons leads to disconnectivity in key cognitive networks and the emergence of symptoms like memory loss. The theory holds that plaques form in the brain many years before clinical symptoms are first observed.[57] Neurofibrillary tangles, consisting of a protein called *tau*, also occur alongside the beta-amyloid plaques. However, it is important to note that research data have *not* clearly demonstrated amyloid reduction slows cog-nitive decline. The assumption that amyloid causes dementia is still an attractive but unproved theory.[58,59]

According to Avramopoulos and associates, "The amyloid hypothesis while exciting at the beginning has not borne the desired fruit of disease-modifying treatments. . . . The treatment development field for Alzheimer's disease is full of tombstones for therapies that failed to show benefit over placebo, and a few instances of therapies that may have worsened the clinical state relative to placebo."[60]

A person typically lives with dementia for 8–10 years from the time of di-agnosis. In its early stages, the individual may be aware of forgetfulness, as

[55] Eric Karran and Bart De Strooper, "The amyloid hypothesis in Alzheimer disease: new insights from new therapeutics," *Nature Reviews Drug Discoveries* 21, no. 4 (April 2022): 306–318, https://doi.org/10.1038/s41573-022-00391-w.

[56] Eric Karran, Marc Mercken, and Bart De Strooper, "The amyloid cascade hypothesis for Alzheimer's disease: An appraisal for the development of therapeutics," *Nature Reviews Drug Discoveries* 10 (August 2011): 698–712, https://doi.org/10.1038/nrd3505.

[57] Willemijn J. Jansen, Rik Ossenkoppele, Dirk L. Knol, et al., and the Amyloid Biomarker Study Group, "Prevalence of cerebral amyloid pathology in persons without dementia: A meta-analysis," *JAMA* 313, no. 19 (May 2015): 1924–1938, doi: 10.1001/jama.2015.4668.

[58] Pam Belluck, "Congressional inquiry into Alzheimer's drug faults its maker and F.D.A.," *New York Times*, accessed December 29, 2022, https://www.nytimes.com/2022/12/29/health/alzheimers-drug-aduhelm-biogen.html?campaign_id=190&emc=edit_ufn_20221229&instance_id=81366&nl=from-the-times&regi_id=63340269&segment_id=121084&te=1&user_id=895343099129dcd1f95fa65a5a136796.

[59] Sarah F. Ackley, Scott C. Zimmerman, Willa D. Brenowitz, et al., "Effect of reductions in am-yloid levels on cognitive change in randomized trials: Instrumental variable meta-analysis," *British Medical Journal* 372, no. 156 (February 2021), doi: 10.1136/bmj.n156. Erratum in: BMJ. 2022 Aug 30;378:o2094. PMID: 33632704; PMCID: PMC7905687.

[60] D. Avramopoulos, D. Kapogiannis, J. M. Leoutsakos, et al., "Developing treatments for Alzheimer's and related disorders with precision medicine: A vision," *Advvances in Experimental Medicine and Biology* 1339 (January 2021): 395–402, doi: 10.1007/978-3-030-78787-5_49. PMID: 35023131; PMCID: PMC9358929.

are family members and friends. In time, the forgetfulness worsens, although people often may retain their older, more distant memories.[61] Several published memoirs offer sensitive glimpses into the lives of those who are affected by these disorders.[62–65]

As dementia slowly advances, the memory problems become more obvious to others, including physicians during clinical examinations. Driving becomes unsafe, and, during this mid-stage, some help is required for daily activities such as cooking and bathing. In the last stage of Alzheimer's, people are no longer be able to care for themselves. Severe personality changes may become manifest; family members are not recognized and patients lose the ability to speak, walk, eat, and drink.

According to a meta-analysis, about one-third of general physicians and half of specialists reported that they usually, regularly, or always *refrain from telling people they have a dementia*.[66] There are several reasons underlying this disturbing finding, including that these are chronic illnesses with bleak prognoses, there are staggeringly terrible social consequences, and giving bad news is an arduous and delicate process requiring sensitivity and time.[67] In addition, limited knowledge or experience in differentiating and dealing with diseases that have cognitive symptoms may lead doctors to be reticent regarding what to say and when to say it.

[61] S. G. Sclan and B. Reisberg, "Functional Assessment Staging (FAST) in Alzheimer's disease: Reliability, validity, and ordinality," *International Psychogeriatrics* 4, Supp. 1 (1992): 55–69, doi: 10.1017/s1041610292001157.

[62] Sandeep Jauhar, *My Father's Brain: Life in the Shadow of Alzheimer's* (New York: Farrar, Straus and Giroux, 2023), 8–13.

[63] Andrew Watson, "Life without memory: Your hippocampus and you: Review of *The Perpetual Now: A Story of Amnesia, Memory, and Love*, by Michael D. Lemonick," accessed June 23, 2023, https://www.learningandthebrain.com/blog/life-without-memory-your-hippocampus-and-you/.

[64] Wendy Mitchell, *Somebody I Used to Know* (New York: Ballantine Books, 2018), 140–141.

[65] Elisabeth Egan, "When her husband said he wanted to die, Amy Bloom listened," *The New York Times*, accessed January 26, 2023, https://www.nytimes.com/2022/03/01/books/review-in-love-memoir-amy-bloom.html.

[66] Lee-Fay Low, Margaret McGrath, Kate Swaffer, and Henry Brodaty, "Communicating a diagnosis of dementia: A systematic mixed studies review of attitudes and practices of health practitioners," *Dementia (London)* 18, no. 7–8 (Oct-Nov 2019, Epub March 2018): 2856–2905, https://pubmed.ncbi.nlm.nih.gov/29544345/.

[67] Robert P. Roca, Susan W. Lehmann, Helen H. Kyomen, James M. Ellison, and Committee on Aging of the Group for the Advancement of Psychiatry, "The science, ethics, and art of disclosing a dementia diagnosis," *The Psychiatric Times*, accessed September 24, 2022, https://www.psychiatrictimes.com/view/the-science-ethics-and-art-of-disclosing-a-dementia-diagnosis.

However, all the above factors are merely rationalizations and excuses. Identification of dementia may not be a simple matter, but it shouldn't be withheld. Patients and families need to start sorting out their futures. Sandy Bem's neuropsychologist was perfectly correct when he immediately advised that she begin "getting her life in order." Dan certainly needed to hear about his dementing illness if he was going to chart out a course of action.

9

For several years prior to Dan's diagnosis, he had been having noticeable difficulty hearing. This led the two men to curtail going to noisy restaurants and crowded social settings. Interestingly, a prospective study has found that mild hearing loss among adults is linked to double the risk of dementia.[1] Moderate loss triples the risk, and people with a severe hearing impairment are five times more likely to develop a dementia. Hearing impairment is cited as being the single most important modifiable risk factor by the Lancet Commission, which focuses on widely available interventions and behaviors to prevent dementing illnesses.[2]

As Dan declared, another of these is exercise. Research suggests that regular moderate to vigorous exercise can promote brain health and reduce the risk of dementia.[3]

Beginning in 2012, some neuroscientists became interested in the potential role of disturbed sleep and how it might interfere with a newly discovered "brain

[1] "The hidden risks of hearing loss," Johns Hopkins Medicine, accessed September 23, 2022, https://www.hopkinsmedicine.org/health/wellness-and-prevention/the-hidden-risks-of-hearing-loss#:~:text=In%20a%20study%20that%20tracked,more%20likely%20to%20develop%20dementia.

[2] Paula Span, "New dementia prevention method may be behavioral, not prescribed," The New York Times, accessed September 23, 2022, https://www.nytimes.com/2022/07/03/health/dementia-treatment-behavior-eye-care.html?action=click&algo=bandit-all-surfaces-variants-shadow-als2-time-cutoff-30&alpha=0.05&block=trending_recirc&fellback=false&imp_id=974790151&impression_id=0b1f5903-fb97-11ec-a0f6-e34bcf3df9d6&index=0&pgtype=Article&pool=pool%2F91fcf81c-4fb0-49ff-bd57-a24647c85ea1&region=footer&req_id=383015720&shadow_implicit2=1.1535746409307759&surface=eos-most-popular-story&variant=3_bandit-eng30s-shadow-als2.

[3] Jianwei Zhu, Fenfen Ge, Yu Zeng, et al., "Physical and mental activity, disease susceptibility, and risk of dementia: A prospective cohort study based on UK Biobank," Neurology 99, no. 8 (August 2022, Epub July 2022): e799–e813, 27;10.1212/WNL. PMID: 35896434. doi: 10.1212/WNL.0000000000200701.

plumbing system" used to flush out broken-down brain cells and other waste materials.[4,5] The so-called *glymphatic fluid* flows through the brain mainly during sleep; it is responsible for clearing out many catabolic products, including the two complex proteins, amyloid-beta and tau, that aggregate and form plaques and tangles. Even among the young and healthy, neurofunction may be affected by sleep deprivation, and the U.S. Department of Defense is funding at least two research projects that have the goal of developing wearable "caps" to improve glymphatic flow during sleep.

Researchers have noted that the risk factors correlating with dementias are similarly mirrored by a condition called *canine cognitive dysfunction*.[6] "Doggy dementia" is found far more often in older dogs who don't get sufficient exercise, as well as in those having impaired hearing and sight. Annette Fitzpatrick, a University of Washington research professor with expertise in dementia in people as well as canines, has commented, "When you don't get stimulation from the outside world, it seems to increase the risk of our not even being able to use our brains as well."[7]

Why did Dan always assume he would be diagnosed with Alzheimer's? The easy answer is that most of us are psychologically predisposed to believe we will suffer the same fate as our parents.[8] If my mother died at a young age, I hold my breath as I approach that birthday. If my father had chronic obstructive pulmonary disease (COPD), then I worry that I will contract the same chronic disorder. Dan watched Wint afflicted by Alzheimer's, and, not surprisingly, he awaited word of the diagnosis from his own physician.

I mention this explanation because while the ultimate cause (or causes) of Alzheimer's disease remains unknown, *genetic factors appear to play only a modest*

[4] "Alzheimer's researchers are studying the brain's plumbing," *The Economist*, accessed October 8, 2022, https://www.economist.com/science-and-technology/alzheimers-researchers-are-studying-the-brains-plumbing/21808465.

[5] Yue Leng, Katie Stone, and Kristine Yaffe, "Race differences in the association between sleep medication use and risk of dementia," *Journal of Alzheimer's Disease* 91, no. 3 (2023): 1133–1139, doi: 10.3233/JAD-221006.

[6] Sarah Yarborough, Annette Fitzpatrick, Stephen M. Schwartz, et al., "Evaluation of cognitive function in the Dog Aging Project: associations with baseline canine characteristics," *Science Reports* 12, no. 13316 (2022), https://doi.org/10.1038/s41598-022-15837-9.

[7] Jan Hoffman, "Will your dog get dementia? A large new study offers clues," *The New York Times*, accessed August 31, 2022, https://www.nytimes.com/2022/08/25/health/dog-dementia-causes.html.

[8] Dawn MacKeen, "'What if this is my destiny?' Children of Alzheimer's patients sometimes fear future diagnosis," *The New York Times*, accessed April 18, 2023, https://www.nytimes.com/2022/08/02/well/mind/alzheimers-caregivers.html?smid=em-share.

role.[9] But, as mentioned, three different genes have been identified that account for the small number of cases of familial, early-onset Alzheimer's. Yet another gene confers some modestly increased risk for the more common late-onset form of the disease; other genes will undoubtably be discovered. The fact that Dan's father had Alzheimer's disease may have been an unfortunate coincidence, and John is confident his husband never took one of the readily available genetic tests, like 23andMe. Even if he had, it's unlikely this would have substantively changed his beliefs or behaviors, although perhaps he could have begun to make death-hastening preparations sooner.

There is an intriguing piece in *The New York Times* describing the misfortune of Chris Hemsworth, best known as "Thor" from the Marvel Universe movies, who has reportedly stepped back from acting after learning he is genetically predisposed to dementia.[10] Ironically, during the previous year, and in a reference to the actor's good-looking parents, another reporter had written, "when it comes to the genetic lottery, [Hemsworth] surely hit the jackpot."[11] But the man who plays the God of Thunder has a grandparent with the disease who no longer can speak coherently or recognize family members.[12] Adding to the irony of his situation, Hemsworth received the genetic test as part of a documentary show about life extension.

Nearly 30 years ago, scientists learned that the APOE gene influences a person's chances of developing Alzheimer's, and there are three variants, each conferring a different risk. People who have the APOE2 variant appear to have a decreased risk; the APOE3 variant neither increases nor decreases risk; and the APOE4 variant signals an increased risk. Individuals inherit one of the APOE

[9] "Causes of Alzheimer's disease: Alzheimer's disease genetics fact sheet," National Institute on Aging, accessed September 22, 2022, https://www.nia.nih.gov/health/alzheimers-disease-genetics-fact-sheet.

[10] Dana G. Smith, "How to know if you have a genetic risk for Alzheimer's," *The New York Times*, accessed November 29, 2022, https://www.nytimes.com/2022/11/23/well/alzheimers-disease-genetic-risk.html.

[11] Maddison Hockey, "Inside Chris, Liam and Luke Hemsworth's wild upbringing with their equally good-looking parents: The three boys weren't always close," Now, accessed November 29, 2022, https://www.nowtolove.com.au/parenting/celebrity-families/chris-hemsworth-parents-67464.

[12] Penelope Clifton, "Chris Hemsworth hasn't seen his grandfather 'in years' after his own shock Alzheimer's prediction: His admission hits home more than ever," kidspot, accessed December 12, 2022, https://www.kidspot.com.au/lifestyle/entertainment/chris-hemsworth-hasnt-seen-his-grandfather-in-years-after-his-own-shock-alzheimers-prediction/news-story/c1a331020ccf635ac7c3be4a2988cc7d.

genes from each parent, and they may play a role in Alzheimer's and related diseases by interfering with brain cell ability to process fats or lipids.[13]

Hemsworth learned that he is unfortunately among the 2–3% of the population who has inherited two copies of the APOE4 gene variant, which is associated with a 30–55% lifetime risk of developing the disease—or, to put it differently, the two copies of the gene confer an eightfold risk of him developing Alzheimer's compared to the general population.[14,15] The 39-year-old told *Vanity Fair* that he hasn't developed any symptoms but wants to focus on mitigating his risk as much as possible.[16]

But having either one or two copies of the APOE4 gene variant *does not inevitably mean a person will get Alzheimer's disease*. The APOE4 gene is only one of many factors contributing to a lifetime risk for developing Alzheimer's disease, and there are numerous people with the dementia who do not have APOE4. This contrasts with another dementing illness, Huntington disease, which is directly caused by a specific gene mutation passed along from a parent.[17] In other words, APOE4 is not a *deterministic* gene, but it is an *indicator* of the likelihood of developing Alzheimer's, as opposed to mutations in the HTT gene that cause Huntington disease.

So how is Chris Hemsworth going to try to reduce his chance of getting Alzheimer's?

Research indicates that those factors which contribute over time to poorer vascular health will increase the risk of dementia.[18] The thinking is that damaged blood vessels in the brain lead to inflammation, the death of neuronal cells, and

[13] Erin Bryant, "Study reveals how APOE4 gene may increase risk for dementia," NIH, accessed April 16, 2023, https://www.nih.gov/news-events/nih-research-matters/study-reveals-how-apoe4-gene-may-increase-risk-dementia.

[14] Carolyn Langlois, Angela Bradbury, Elisabeth M. Wood, et al., "Alzheimer's prevention initiative generation program: Development of an APOE genetic counseling and disclosure process in the context of clinical trials," *Alzheimers Dement (N Y)* 5 (November 2019): 705–716, doi: 10.1016/j.trci.2019.09.013. PMID: 31921963; PMCID: PMC6944715.

[15] Sandeep Jauhar, *My Father's Brain: Life in the Shadow of Alzheimer's* (New York: Farrar, Straus and Giroux, 2023), 52.

[16] Anthony Breznican, "Chris Hemsworth changed his life after an ominous health warning," Vanity Fair, accessed April 16, 2023, https://www.vanityfair.com/hollywood/2022/11/chris-hemsworth-exclusive-interview-alzheimers-limitless.

[17] "Huntington disease," Medline Plus, accessed April 16, 2023, https://medlineplus.gov/genetics/condition/huntington-disease/#:~:text=Mutations%20in%20the%20HTT%20gene,making%20a%20protein%20called%20huntingtin.

[18] John Mamo, "Chris Hemsworth's Alzheimer's gene doesn't guarantee he'll develop dementia. Here's what we can all do to reduce our risk," The Conversation, accessed December 7, 2022, https://theconversation.com/chris-hemsworths-alzheimers-gene-doesnt-guarantee-hell-develop-dementia-heres-what-we-can-all-do-to-reduce-our-risk-195094#:~:text=Chris%20Hemsworth%2C%20famous%20for%20his,for%20Alzheimer's%202%2D3%20times.

cognitive impairment. Accordingly, clinicians recommend several well-known healthy habits, including the previously mentioned exercise, getting sufficient sleep, and attending to hearing loss, but also more rigorously controlling high blood pressure, paying attention to nutrition, remaining socially engaged, and curbing excessive alcohol consumption.

As for treatment? While a recent article rejoices that, "Suddenly, it looks like we're in a golden age for medicine,"[19] this hardly appears to be the dementia story. When Dan investigated the topic, he discovered that there hadn't been a new Alzheimer's therapy in nearly two decades. Dr. Khachaturian, the editor-in-chief of the journal *Alzheimer's & Dementia*, entitled a speech "40 years of Alzheimer's research failure: Now what?"[20] Among the points he made is that while there are currently five approved medications (which according to Dr. Macchi have just jumped to seven) to address the worsening of cognitive and memory symptoms, they are at best modestly effective in only *some* individuals for a *limited* time.[21] Medications like donepezil (sold under the brand name Aricept, among others) "do nothing to slow or reverse the progression of the disease" and are marketed with the inscrutable instructions that they should be stopped if no benefit is seen.[22] Neurologist Dr. Gregory Day has been quoted as saying "I'm sure you're aware that none of our disease-modifying medications works one bit in people who already have symptoms. If we wait till people have dementia, the freight train has left the station, and we can't slow it down. Anyone who says they can is lying or trying to make money off of you."[23]

Why? Because Alzheimer's disease is actually a heterogeneous clinical entity and not a single disorder, it is triggered by multiple biological processes, and, as stated earlier, there may be a lengthy asymptomatic or preclinical stage preceding MCI. Some research suggests there is a 20- to 30-year interval between the first appearance of amyloid positivity and the onset of dementia.[24]

[19] D. Wallace-Wells, "Suddenly, it looks like we're in a golden age for medicine," *The New York Times,* June 23, 2023, https://www.nytimes.com/2023/06/23/magazine/golden-age-medicine-bio medical-innovation.html.

[20] Zaven S. Khachaturian, "40 years of Alzheimer's research failure: Now what? Decades-long odyssey with little to show," MedPage Today, accessed October 8, 2022, https://www.medpagetoday.com/neurology/alzheimersdisease/75075.

[21] Alzheimer's Association, "2014 Alzheimer's disease facts and figures," *Alzheimer & Dementia* 10, no. 2 (2014): e47–e92.

[22] Jauhar, *My Father's Brain*, 94.

[23] Ibid.,148.

[24] Willemijn J. Jansen, Rik Ossenkoppele, Dirk L. Knol, et al., "Prevalence of cerebral amyloid pathology in persons without dementia," *JAMA* 313, no. 19 (2015): 1924–1938, doi: 10.1001/jama.2015.4668.

Both the preclinical stage and the different etiological factors need to be the foci of therapeutic efforts.

Another contributor to this complex situation is a group of older people who complain of suffering from worsening memory and cognition but are not found to have objective impairments or deterioration on neuropsychological testing.[25] Labeled as *subjective cognitive decline*, long-term follow-up investigations have found them to be twice as likely to develop dementia as individuals without this condition.

In November of 2020, a new drug, aducanumab, faced an examination by a federal panel of experts from the Food and Drug Administration (FDA), and it was rejected as being potentially unsafe and only marginally beneficial.[26,27,28,29] Later, in June 2021, this same medication was granted conditional approval by the FDA following intensive campaigning by families and representatives from dementia advocacy groups who desperately wanted a therapy.[30] They asked unanswerable questions: How far should we go when the alternative for our loved one is inexorable deterioration and death? What is sacrificed in the process?[31]

Their response was that the FDA *must* support the release of aducanumab. Marketed as Aduhelm, the intravenous infusion of this medication was priced by its manufacturer, Biogen, at $56,000 a year.

Three members of the federal panel were sufficiently upset with the drug's authorization that they resigned. Dr. Aaron Kesselheim wrote that the FDA's move was "probably the worst drug approval decision in recent

---

[25] A. J. Mitchell, H. Beaumont, D. Ferguson, M. Yadegarfar, and B. Stubbs, "Risk of dementia and mild cognitive impairment in older people with subjective memory complaints: Meta-analysis," *Acta Psychiatrica Scandinavica* 130, no. 6 (December 2014): 439–451, https://doi.org/10.1111/acps.12336.

[26] G. Caleb Alexander, David S. Knopman, Scott S. Emerson, et al., "Revisiting FDA approval of aducanumab," *New England Journal of Medicine* 385 (2021): 769–771.

[27] P. Belluck, S. Kaplan, and R. Robbins, "How an unproven Alzheimer's drug got approved," *The New York Times*, July 19, 2021, accessed September 23, 2022, https://www.nytimes.com/2021/07/19/health/alzheimers-drug-aduhelm-FDA.

[28] D. S. Knopman, D. T. Jones, and M. D. Greicius, "Failure to demonstrate efficacy of aducanumab: an analysis of the EMERGE and ENGAGE trials as reported by Biogen, December 2019," *Alzheimers & Dementia* 17 (2021): 696–701.

[29] A. J. Mitchell, H. Beaumont, D. Ferguson, M. Yadegarfar, and B. Stubbs, "Risk of dementia and mild cognitive impairment in older people with subjective memory complaints: Meta-analysis," *Acta Psychiatrica Scandinavica* 130, no. 6 (December 2014): 439–451, https://doi.org/10.1111/acps.12336.

[30] A. Bateman-House, "How to make experimental treatment less of a gamble," *The New York Times*, October 14, 2022, accessed October 15, 2022, https://www.nytimes.com/2022/10/14/opinion/experimental-treatment.html.

[31] D. J. Lamas, "How far do you go when the alternative is death?" May 12, 2022, accessed October 15, 2022, https://www.nytimes.com/2022/05/12/opinion/terminal-illness-clinical-trials-drugs-FDA.html?action=click&module=RelatedLinks&pgtype=Article.

U.S. history."[32] Subsequently, the agency walked back its assessment and is now only recommending use by patients with mild memory and cognitive problems. A Congressional inquiry has found that the FDA's approval process for aducanumab was "rife with irregularities," and it has criticized Biogen for setting an "unjustifiably high price."[33]

This was followed shortly thereafter by the failure of another drug, crenezumab, in a decade-long clinical trial to prevent or slow cognitive decline in a sample of people genetically destined to develop Alzheimer's disease.[34] That study did not show any significant benefit and was halted.

As of September 2022, there were still 143 drugs in development spread across 172 clinical trials.[35] And while Biogen now has less confidence in aducanumab and crenezumab, and the company has parted ways with its CEO, a business website headline that followed these developments went on to proclaim, "It's time for lecanemab!"[36]

In January of 2023, the FDA initially approved this new monoclonal antibody for use in early and mild stages of Alzheimer's disease, and, in July, it gave full approval of the drug for patients.[37-39] The research data remain unclear as

[32] N. P. Taylor, "Harvard's Kesselheim quits AdComm over FDA's Aduhelm approval," Fierce Biotech, June 11, 2021, https://www.fiercebiotech.com/biotech/harvard-s-kesselheim-quits-adcomm-over-FDA-s-aduhelm-approval.

[33] Pam Belluck, "Congressional inquiry into Alzheimer's drug faults its maker and FDA," *The New York Times*, accessed December 29, 2022, https://www.nytimes.com/2022/12/29/health/alzheimers-drug-aduhelm-biogen.html?campaign_id=190&emc=edit_ufn_20221229&instance_id=81366&nl=from-the-times&regi_id=63340269&segment_id=121084&te=1&user_id=89534 3099129dcd1f95fa65a5a136796.

[34] Pam Belluck, "Trial of new Alzheimer's drug reports disappointing results," *The New York Times*, accessed September 23, 2022, https://www.nytimes.com/2022/06/16/health/alzheimers-drug-crenezumab.html.

[35] A. Armstrong, "Beyond headlines and amyloid, the Alzheimer's pipeline chugs along," Fierce Biotech, September 1, 2022, accessed September 26, 2022, https://www.fiercebiotech.com/biotech/beyond-headlines-and-amyloid-alzheimers-pipeline-chugs-along..

[36] Annalee Armstrong, "Biogen shoves Aduhelm to the side: It's time for lecanemab," Fierce Biotech, accessed September 25, 2022, https://www.fiercebiotech.com/biotech/biogen-shoves-aduhelm-side-its-time-lecanemab.

[37] Brenda Goodman, "After promising data, experts say many questions remain over an experimental Alzheimer's drug," CTV News, accessed December 4, 2022, https://www.ctvnews.ca/health/after-promising-data-experts-say-many-questions-remain-over-an-experimental-alzheimer-s-drug-1.6095240.

[38] Meredith Cohn, "NIH expands faster path used to develop COVID-19 screening to tests, therapies for Alzheimer's and other neurological disorders," *The Baltimore Sun*, accessed October 17, 2022, https://www.baltimoresun.com/health/bs-hs-neurological-disorders-incubator-20221017-ltod7eusrna4pb2pkzvaihutv4-story.html.

[39] "A drug for Alzheimer's disease that seems to work: It is not perfect. And it has side-effects. But it may be the real deal," *The Economist*, accessed December 7, 2022, https://www.economist.com/scie

to whether the drug (marketed as Leqembi) can slow cognitive decline enough that any changes are noticeable to patients and families.[40] Total treatment costs could run to about $90,000 annually, including medical visits and required regular brain scans; Medicare will presumably cover 80% of the medication cost for eligible patients.[41–43]

The FDA's decision marks the first time in two decades that a drug for Alzheimer's has received full approval, but the agency also added a black-box warning on the drug's label, stating that it can cause "serious and life-threatening events," and there were fatalities among the research subjects. The panel has explicitly stated that lecanemab cannot repair cognitive damage, reverse the course of the disease, or stop it from worsening.

Donanemab, Lilly's new investigational medicine, works in the same way as lecanemab, through an amyloid-targeting antibody therapy.[44] While neither of these drugs purports to be a cure, a multinational collaborative study of donanemab has demonstrated that it can alter the course of disease—slow down the rate at which memory and thinking skills decline—among patients with Alzheimer's-related MCI.[45] In a sample involving 1,736 participants, the

nce-and-technology/2022/11/30/a-drug-for-alzheimers-disease-that-seems-to-work?utm_cont ent=article-link-5&etear=nl_today_5&utm_campaign=r.the-economist-today&utm_medium= email.internal-newsletter.np&utm_source=salesforce-marketing-cloud&utm_term=11/30/ 2022&utm_id=1406016.

[40] Pam Belluck, "FDA Approves new treatment for early Alzheimer's," *The New York Times*, accessed January 10, 2023, https://www.nytimes.com/2023/01/06/health/alzheimers-drug-leqe mbi-lecanemab.html?campaign_id=190&emc=edit_ufn_20230106&instance_id=82078&nl= from-the-times&regi_id=63340269&segment_id=121829&te=1&user_id=895343099129dcd1f 95fa65a5a136796.

[41] Pam Belluck, "New federal decisions make Alzheimer's drug leqembi widely accessible," *The New York Times*, accessed July 6, 2023, https://www.nytimes.com/2023/07/06/health/alzheimers-leqembi-medicare.html.

[42] "Alzheimer's Association welcomes U.S. FDA approval of lecanemab," Alzheimer's Association, accessed January 10, 2023, https://www.alz.org/news/2023/lecanemab-FDA-approved.

[43] Gina Kolata and Francesca Paris, "The medicine is a miracle, but only if you can afford it: A wave of new treatments have cured devastating diseases. When the costs are too much, even for the insured, patients hunt for other ways to pay," *The New York Times*, accessed February 7, 2023, https://www.nytimes.com/2023/02/07/health/medicine-insurance-payments.html?campaign_ id=34&emc=edit_sc_20230207&instance_id=84696&nl=science-times&regi_id=63340269&seg ment_id=124649&te=1&user_id=895343099129dcd1f95fa65a5a136796.

[44] Mark A. Mintun, Albert C. Lo, Cynthia Duggan Evans, et al., "Donanemab in early Alzheimer's disease," *New England Journal of Medicine* 384, no. 18 (May 2021): 1691–1704, doi: 10.1056/ NEJMoa2100708.

[45] John R. Sims, Jennifer A. Zimmer, Cynthia D. Evans, et al., "Donanemab in early symptomatic Alzheimer disease: The TRAILBLAZER-ALZ 2 randomized clinical trial," *JAMA* 330, no. 6 (2023): 512–527, doi: 10.1001/jama.2023.13239.

disease process appears to have been decelerated and the clinical progression was significantly slowed at the 76-week point.

According to geriatric psychiatrist, Dr. Brent Forester (July 13, 2023, email), the Chair of Psychiatry at Tufts University School of Medicine, "The advent of monoclonal antibody therapies holds out the promise to more effectively address the cognitive and functional decline associated with dementia by enhancing the removal of beta amyloid from the brain. However, our current healthcare systems do not have the infrastructure needed to identify appropriate individuals who may benefit from these therapies, including, in particular, individuals from underserved populations."

Dr. Forester further emphasizes: "In addition to biological therapies, the approach to dementia care must be holistic, taking into account not only the cognitive and functional aspects of dementia but also the behavioral and psychological symptoms. Behavioral symptoms drive the burden of illness for patients and their care partners. Integrated, holistic, collaborative models of dementia care are a cost-effective approach to timely diagnosis and address behavioral and psychological symptoms of dementia, support family care partners, and lower the total cost of healthcare for this population."

*****

Over the past few decades, deep brain stimulation (DBS) has been explored as an alternative or adjunct for the medication management of Parkinson's disease, and this has also led to it being tried for mild Alzheimer's disease.[46,47] DBS is a surgical treatment that modifies the irregular neuronal activity of the target region of the brain via electrical stimulation through surgically placed electrical leads. Research examining its effects on memory and cognition have focused on the fornix, a fiber bundle that carries approximately 1.2 million axons and constitutes the major projection linking various nodes within the circuit of Papez. DBS has been found to drive brain electrical activity throughout this circuit and to increase glucose metabolism in temporal and parietal areas after 12 months, in contrast to the progressive decrease in metabolism that commonly occurs in Alzheimer's. In a Phase II study, there were no overall differences in cognitive outcomes for participants; however, the subgroup of participants aged 65 and

[46] Chantelle Lachance, Carolyn Spry, and Danielle MacDougall, "Deep brain stimulation for Parkinson's disease: A review of clinical effectiveness, cost-effectiveness, and guidelines," Ottawa: Canadian Agency for Drugs and Technologies in Health, accessed March 25, 2023, https://www.ncbi.nlm.nih.gov/books/NBK538348/.

[47] Michael S. Okun, "Deep-brain stimulation for Parkinson's disease," *New England Journal of Medicine* 367, no. 16 (October 2012): 1529–1538, doi: 10.1056/NEJMct1208070.

older may have derived some benefit. On the other hand, the study found a possible worsening in patients younger than 65.[48]

Finally, in what a medical geneticist is calling "a Hail Mary treatment idea for Alzheimer's," an investigatory team is exploring the effect of using a virus injected into the spinal fluid to flood research subjects with APOE2.[49] The plan is to convert the brain milieu of individuals who have two APOE4 variants (like Chris Hemsworth) into that of people with a single APOE4 and a single APOE2. The hope is that this will possibly slice their Alzheimer's risk in half.

Yet another research group is exploring the use of gene editing, a newer technology that does not rely on a virus but instead uses the molecular machine, CRISPR, to insert a protective gene. For diseases other than dementias there are now four novel gene therapies, and pharmaceutical companies are charging patients between $2.1 million and $3.5 million to receive each of them.[50-52]

*****

I am convinced that Dan, like columnist Michael Kinsley, offers us a foretaste of the imminent future.[53] Kinsley was 43 when diagnosed with Parkinson's. He has written that he feels, "like a scout from my generation, sent out ahead to experience in my fifties what even the healthiest boomers are going to experience

---

[48] Andres M. Lozano, Lisa Fosdick, M. Mallar Chakravarty, et al, "A Phase II study of fornix deep brain stimulation in mild Alzheimer's disease," *Journal of Alzheimers Disease* 54, no. 2 (September 2016): 777–787. doi: 10.3233/JAD-160017. PMID: 27567810; PMCID: PMC5026133.

[49] Gina Kolata, "A promising trial targets a genetic risk for Alzheimer's: Preliminary results offer hope that gene therapy can protect people with a version of the brain disease driven by a particular gene variant," *The New York Times*, accessed December 5, 2022, https://www.nytimes.com/2022/12/02/health/alzheimers-apoe4-gene-therapy.html?smid=em-share.

[50] Fyodor Urnov, "We can cure disease by editing a person's DNA. Why aren't we?," *The New York Times*, accessed December 9, 2022, https://www.nytimes.com/2022/12/09/opinion/crispr-gene-editing-cures.html.

[51] Allison DeAngelis, "As gene-editing moves mainstream, a pioneer in the field is testing whether it could prevent Alzheimer's," Insider, accessed December 9, 2022, https://www.businessinsider.com/gene-editing-pioneer-david-liu-developing-drug-to-prevent-alzheimers-2021-11.

[52] Ananya Bhattacharya, "A hemophilia drug that just won FDA approval pegs a one-time $3.5 million vial against several millions in lifelong costs: The most expensive drugs in the US are gene therapy ones that alter DNA to cure disease," Quartz, accessed December 12, 2022, https://qz.com/a-hemophilia-drug-that-just-won-FDA-approval-pegs-a-one-1849820064.

[53] Phillip Lopate, "Michael Kinsley's 'Old Age: A Beginner's Guide,'" *The New York Times*, accessed September 22, 2022, https://www.nytimes.com/2016/04/24/books/review/michael-kinsley-old-age-a-beginners-guide.html?ref=todayspaper.

in the sixties, seventies, or eighties." Kinsley's glimpse at what lies ahead is undeniably worrisome: "Of the 79 million boomers," he explains, "28 million are expected to develop Alzheimer's or some other form of dementia. . . . That adds up to about 35%, or one out of three." As for those hopeful individuals who seek to avoid a dire future by jogging daily or eating products derived from jelly fish . . . Kinsley declares, "They will get Alzheimer's anyway."

10

Is it fair to say that Dan intended to commit *suicide*?

In an essay adapted from her classic book on the subject, Professor of Philosophy and Medical Ethics from the University of Utah Medical School Margaret Pabst Battin offers the most lucid answer to this issue.[1,2] She begins by inquiring, "What makes something suicide? Is it about causation . . . or is it about intention?" Professor Battin concludes, "This duality explains much of the way we label life-ending acts: when we focus on *mechanism* we call them suicide, but when we focus on *intention* we give those of which we approve of the intention much more favorable labels."

If one emphasizes Dan's intention—to curtail the suffering engendered by his brain disease—and if one believes that this is acceptable, then the word "suicide" does not fit.[3] By contrast, if one focuses on the mechanism of Dan's plan—the ingestion of a large quantity of pills expressly for the purpose of ending life—then it might understandably be labeled as a suicide.

Professor Battin points out (June 1, 2020, interview) that "it is the very existence of modern medicine that has given rise to the dilemma of whether to endure the very, very long downhill slope that may lead to what can be a difficult death or take earlier steps to bring our lives to an easier end. This is a personal and societal choice to be taken reflectively, not decided in advance on the basis of slanted language."

And by slanted language, she means emotionally powerful words like suicide.

---

[1] Margaret Pabst Battin, "'Death with dignity': Is it suicide?," OUP Blog, accessed May 29, 2023, https://blog.oup.com/2015/11/death-with-dignity-suicide/.

[2] Margaret Pabst Battin, *The Ethics of Suicide: Historical Sources* (New York: Oxford University Press, 2015).

[3] Rachel E. Gross, "How aid in dying became medical, not moral: The debate over aid in dying still rages in the language that medicine and the media use to describe the practice," *The New York Times*, accessed October 24, 2023, https://www.nytimes.com/2023/10/24/science/medical-dying-suicide.html.

Rebecca Brown, the director of New Hampshire Alliance for End of Life Options, emphasizes that patients who wish for assisted or accelerated dying—like Dan—would ideally prefer to extend their meaningful lives, but "death has chosen them."[4] Their personalities will dissolve, and they are going to physically deteriorate regardless of their wishes, and it is only a matter of time when this will occur.[5] To foreshorten life, whether by taking an overdose, refusing life-prolonging treatments, or requesting terminal sedation, etc., may qualify as the least bad option.[6]

On the other hand, the Center for Disease Control and Prevention has an exceedingly broad definition of suicide as being a "death caused by injuring oneself with the intent to die."[7] This echoes the definition in 1897 of Émile Durkheim, an eminent French sociologist, who described it as a "death resulting directly or indirectly from a positive or negative act of the victim himself, which he knows will produce this result."[8,9]

John and I directly associate suicide with hopelessness and psychopathology; neither of us considered Dan's wish to end his life as being a product of irrationality, major depression, or other psychiatric disorders. On rare occasions, Dan used "suicide" to describe what he intended to do, but he didn't especially care for the word; more often, he relied on descriptive expressions such as "pharmaceutical overdose."

I found it interesting that during the webcast of Compassion & Choice (C&C) and the American Society on Aging, Dan intentionally omitted revealing any wish on his part to kill himself. He explained to me that neither sponsoring organization wanted to be identified with such a decision—however it was labeled.

The C&C Toolkit focuses on the need for completing "dementia directives" before the illness begins to substantially sap one's mental acuity, and it emphasizes

[4] Michelle Liu and Julia Furukawa, "Vermont now allows people from other states to use its medical aid in dying law: What will that mean for NH?," New Hampshire Public Radio, accessed May 13, 2023, https://www.nhpr.org/nh-news/2023-05-12/vermont-now-allows-people-from-other-states-to-use-its-medical-aid-in-dying-law-what-will-that-mean-for-nh.

[5] Tom Preston, *Patient-Directed Dying: A Call for Legalized Aid in Dying for the Terminally Ill* (Lincoln, NE: iUniverse, Inc., 2006), xviii.

[6] John Michael Bostwick and Lewis M. Cohen, "Differentiating suicide from life-ending acts and end-of-life decisions: A model based on chronic kidney disease and dialysis," *Psychosomatics* 50, no. 1 (2009): 1–7, https//:doi.org/10.1176/appi.psy.50.1.1.

[7] "Facts about suicide," Center for Disease Control and Prevention, accessed October 9, 2022, https://www.cdc.gov/suicide/facts/index.html.

[8] W. S. F. Pickering and Geoffrey Walford; British Centre for Durkheimian Studies, *Durkheim's Suicide: A Century of Research and Debate* (London and New York: Psychology Press & Routledge Classic Editions, 2000), 25.

[9] "Suicide (Durkheim book)," Wikipedia, accessed April 21, 2023, https://en.wikipedia.org/wiki/Suicide_(Durkheim_book).

the existence of what it calls "natural exit ramps." The latter include refusal of hospitalizations, non-resuscitation upon request, and refraining from artificial nutrition and hydration with feeding tubes or persistent spoon feeding.[10] For people, like Dan, who wished to truncate dementia, one might add to this list the cessation of all future cancer-screening procedures, such as colonoscopies and PSA blood tests, as well as the avoidance of cardiac stress exams, pacemakers, and implantable defibrillators. Likewise, one might consider declining antibiotics in the event of infections, annual flu vaccines, and almost everything that doesn't directly entail symptom amelioration.

Considerable assertiveness is required on the part of people who wish to withhold or withdraw such medical treatments since many medical professionals are often disinclined to even participate in these conversations or support the decisions. Whether it is a concern on the part of clinicians that they are not accused of ageism, the wish by some family members that their loved ones receive every possible therapy, the idiosyncratic financial incentives in American medicine, or just plain inertia, the elderly—and people with dementing illnesses—are often started on and continue to receive unwise and sometimes extremely aggressive treatments.

How unwise and how aggressive?

Alvin (Woody) H. Moss, MD, Professor of Nephrology at West Virginia University School of Medicine, has published extensively (email October 9, 2022) about the enormous numbers of older Americans with dementia and kidney failure who are begun on chronic maintenance dialysis. This occurs despite (1) research showing they may not live any longer with dialysis than without it, (2) they are more likely to have dialysis complications, (3) dialysis centers are in many respects "dementia-unfriendly" environments, (4) people who have dementias may not be able to cooperate safely with the dialysis process, and (5) they often experience a significant decline in cognitive function after initiating the kidney replacement therapy.[11] However, according to Dr. Moss, "Nephrologists are more comfortable starting patients on dialysis than withholding it [because they mistakenly] equate not offering dialysis with 'no care.' "

The C&C Toolkit refrains from directly addressing any patient or family desire to control the method and timing of death more actively. It certainly does

---

[10] C. A. Meier and Thuan D. Ong, "To feed or not to feed? A case report and ethical analysis of withholding food and drink in a patient with advanced dementia," *Journal of Pain and Symptom Management* 50, no. 6 (2015): 887–890.

[11] C. S. Kart, "In the matter of Earle Spring: Some thoughts on one court's approach to senility," *The Gerontologist* 21, no. 4 (August 1981): 417–423, https://doi.org/10.1093/geront/21.4.417

not mention the word "suicide," which many authorities would be quick to label as the ultimate "unnatural exit ramp."[12]

By contrast, Dan was always frank with friends, family, and even casual acquaintances about his wish to take an overdose. But he appreciated the unstated needs of the American Society on Aging and C&C, and he chose not to publicly spar with either nonprofit organization over this issue.

*****

From the beginning, Dan and I tried to keep our relationship as clear as possible. He understood that while I was a physician, I had solely approached him in my capacity as an author. Every phone contact was begun by my explicitly seeking his consent to record the interview as part of this writing project.

Neither John nor Dan was particularly interested in peppering me with questions about my own life. It sufficed that they had conducted a Google search and read my previous book. In addition, Dan had already established his own network of medical professionals and right-to-die advocates; he didn't require specific advice from me. When occasionally tempted to offer a suggestion or otherwise intervene, I generally demurred, confident that the two men were already collaborating with knowledgeable people on every step of the journey.

Nevertheless, I was always aware of the moral quandaries implicit in this endeavor. Chief among these was that I had chosen to bear witness—as a journalist—to a man's desire to die. I knew fully well that many would view Dan's death as a suicide—even if John and I didn't. What's more, I did not intend to interfere. It required a fair amount of soul-searching to admit that I wanted him to succeed.

William S. Breitbart, MD, the Jimmie C. Holland Chair in Psychiatric Oncology at Memorial Sloan Kettering Cancer Center in New York, has intellectually struggled over similar bioethical issues with his patients who suffer from cancer. Dr. Breitbart generally celebrates mankind's drive to survive under adversity, and he is quick to quote Camus, Kierkegaard, and Viktor Frankl.[13] However, he occasionally encounters people, like Dan, who exemplify the Shakespearean dilemma, "To be or not to be? That is the question!" or who espouse the Duke of York's proclamation, "Though death be poor, it ends a mortal woe."[14] Dr. Breitbart characterized Dan as "a human being taking the existential

---

[12] Kathleen M. Foley and Herbert Hendin, *The Case Against Assisted Suicide: For the Right to End-of-Life Care* (Baltimore, MD: Johns Hopkins University Press, 2002).

[13] Viktor E. Frankl, *Man's Search for Ultimate Meaning* (New York: Perseus Publishing, 2000).

[14] William Shakespeare, *Richard II*. Barbara Mowat, Paul Werstine, Michael Poston, and Rebecca Niles, eds. (Washington DC: Folger Shakespeare Library, n.d.), accessed August 16, 2023, https://www.folger.edu/explore/shakespeares-works/richard-ii/read/2/1/.

responsibility of deciding whether one's meaningful life was now over." The veteran psycho-oncologist didn't envy me my role as a journalist in this situation.

*****

Early in our series of interviews, Dan brought up the subject of *Still Alice*, an award-winning 2014 film based on the novel by Lisa Genova.[15] In the movie, Julianne Moore is a linguist diagnosed with early-onset dementia. The plot depicts not only the way the disease inexorably takes control of Alice's life, but also how any wish on her part to abbreviate existence becomes nearly impossible.

In an interview, Dan alluded to an especially heartbreaking scene where Alice discovers a video she had previously made for herself. Anticipating that her Alzheimer's disease was going to progress, the woman gave simple instructions in the video about how to take out a hidden bottle of sleeping pills from the drawer and use them to overdose. But by the time she watches it, Alice is already too impaired to carry out her own directions. She is distracted, accidentally spills the tablets all over the floor, and then entirely forgets what she is trying to do.

When Dan and I each separately watched the movie, both of us had the same reaction: we wanted to shout at her to pick up the pills, turn the video back on, and try once again.

Dan desperately feared the consequences of procrastinating. During our phone call, his voice cracked as he said, "There are so many things Alice could have done . . . she needed to tell more people, and she needed to ask more from her loved ones, so they would alert her as to the right time."

Realistically, I didn't think any of those were especially satisfactory solutions to Alice's predicament. But he and I both felt abysmal at what lay ahead in the future for this fictional character whose memory and executive functions were disintegrating. However, in the novel's final scene, she appears to still enjoy walking in the park with a caretaker, holding her grandchild, and being kissed by her daughter. At the same time, Alice is barely able to speak, doesn't know where she is sitting, and is incapable of recognizing loved ones.

Alice may have been a make-believe character, but she felt as real to us as Sandy Bem, which is a testament to Genova's skillfulness as a novelist and the background research she conducted. From our perspective, Alice failed by waiting too long; Sandy succeeded by actively fulfilling her plan to die on time.

During my many interviews with Dan, and as especially when I thought about suicide, I frequently wondered, *Was I wandering barefoot through a verdant meadow while deluding myself that there weren't any thorns or poison ivy underfoot?*

[15] "Still Alice (novel)," Wikipedia, accessed September 23, 2022, https://en.wikipedia.org/wiki/Still_Alice_(novel).

Was there a more ethically correct path for me to follow as a journalist and as a human being?

Concerning which my friend, Harvey Chochinov, MD, PhD, Distinguished Professor of Psychiatry at the University of Manitoba, who, like Dr. Breitbart, is a thoughtful and adamant opponent of medical aid in dying (MAiD),[16] wrote (October 22, 2022, email): "Lew, I think if your feet, metaphorically, weren't so itchy and oozing blood, you wouldn't be asking the questions."

[16] Harvey Max Chochinov, "The platinum rule: A new standard for person-centered care," *Journal of Palliative Medicine* 25, no. 6 (June 2022; Epub February 2022): 854–856, doi: 10.1089/jpm.2022.0075.

11

Barking could be heard in the background when I next connected with Dan. "What's that?" I asked.

"My dog, Friday," he responded. "We're just back from a walk and she's still stirred up. I think there's a bird by our window."

"So, what's on your mind today?" I inquired.

It turned out that Dan was stirred up, too, and he wanted to discuss his ineligibility to receive medical assistance in dying (MAiD). The conversation also veered back into a discussion of whether "suicide" was the correct word for his intention to accelerate his demise.

The Kansas native had originally moved to Oregon partly because of his admiration for its death-with-dignity law. This was the first such in the United States, and there are now 10 other jurisdictions—including California, Colorado, the District of Columbia, Hawaii, Maine, New Jersey, Montana, New Mexico, Vermont, and Washington—that have each modeled their end-of-life care acts and clinical protocols around Oregon's 26-year-old statute. Every year additional states try to pass similar laws or tweak and improve existing ones. But, in common, they all currently exclude people who have dementias, and they offer a challenge to how our society defines suicide.

The first of these matters was of practical concern to Dan and other people with dementing illnesses. The second is more problematic for bioethicists, theologians, clinicians, and psychiatrists like me, but it also factors in on how family and ordinary people might view Dan's wish to hasten his death.

Dementia was excluded by Oregon's requirements that qualifying patients be of sound mind—that is, have "capacity" (defined as being able to make and communicate healthcare decisions)—and have a prognosis of death within 6 months.[1]

---

[1] "Death with Dignity Act requirements," Oregon Health Authority, accessed April 21, 2023, https://www.oregon.gov/oha/PH/PROVIDERPARTNERRESOURCES/EVALUATIONRESEARCH/DEATHWITHDIGNITYACT/Documents/requirements.pdf.

Dan was aware that Alzheimer's disease often takes decades—not 6 months—before it kills people. In addition, because it primarily affects memory and cognition, one's competence or capacity can potentially be challenged even in its earliest stages.[2] Author Katie Engelhart has correctly written: "Many adult children are surprised to learn that a diagnosis of dementia, on its own, does *not* disqualify a parent from making big decisions. The adult child assumes that the first pronouncement from a doctor . . . immediately flips some kind of decisional switch, rendering the parent incompetent to choose."[3]

But Engelhart continues: "Within medicine, there is no such switch. To an informed clinician, patients are never 'capable' or 'incapable' in a global sense. Instead, they are capable or incapable of making a specific decision, in a specific context, at a specific moment. In practice, this means that a person with dementia might retain what doctors call 'decision-making capacity' for years and then lose it in stages: the complex choices first, the simple ones later. She might, for instance, lose the capacity to choose among treatment options but retain the capacity to decide which family member should make the decision for her. In each case, the firm bioethical consensus is that we should err on the side of assuming capacity. A person is capable until proved otherwise, even if she has dementia."

In other words, the mere fact that a person carries a diagnosis of Alzheimer's or of Lewy body disease or, for that matter, paranoid schizophrenia, does not mean the individual lacks capacity. There is an assumption in medicine and in the law that people retain this unless proven otherwise.[4] Engelhart is correct that even when a patient lacks capacity for one type of medical decision, this also does not mean that they lack capacity for all medical decisions.[5] However, when it comes to the American end-of-life care acts and clinical protocols, capacity (and competency) are often automatically and incorrectly called into question for people who have dementing illnesses.

[2] Harvey M. Chochinov and Leonard Schwartz, "Depression and the Will to Live in Terminally Ill Patients," in Kathleen Foley and Herbert Hendin (eds.), *The Case Against Assisted Suicide: For the Right to End-of-Life Care* (Baltimore: Johns Hopkins University Press, 2002), 266–267.

[3] Katie Engelhart, "The mother who changed: A story of dementia," *The New York Times Magazine*, accessed May 10, 2023, https://www.nytimes.com/2023/05/09/magazine/dementia-mother.html.

[4] Robert A. Burt, *Taking Care of Strangers: The Rule of Law in Doctor-Patient Relations* (New York and London: Free Press/Collier Macmillan, 1979).

[5] Linda Ganzini, Ladislav Volicer, William Nelson, and Arthur Derse, "Pitfalls in assessment of decision-making capacity," *Psychosomatics* 44, no. 3 (May-June 2003): 237–243, doi: 10.1176/appi.psy.44.3.237. PMID: 12724505.

Competency is a legal term determined by a judge, which describes a person's ability to participate in legal processes.[6,7] By contrast, *capacity* is determined by a physician, and it refers to a patient's ability to make autonomous decisions regarding their care.[8,9] Psychiatric consultants, like me, follow capacity guidelines and rely mainly on four standards for assessing decision-making: Does the individual understand relevant information, appreciate the situation by being able to rationally manipulate the information, arrive at a conclusion, and communicate their choice?[10,11] Psychiatrists rarely employ standardized capacity instruments like the MacArthur Competence Assessment Tool for Clinical Research (MacCAT-CR).[12] This has been translated into several languages and is the best validated questionnaire, but it is time-consuming, difficult to use, and relegated to research purposes.

As long as I'm defining some concepts, I also want to mention *bioethics*, which is the philosophical study of controversies engendered by advances in medicine and technology. Bioethicists explore the relationship between medical practice, theology, law, politics, and other intersecting bodies of knowledge.

*****

Dan said with considerable feeling, "I'm willing to talk to you and have my story published because I'm furious that I can't take part in a state-wide program—Death with Dignity—that I think would make it easier for my family and me."

[6] Stanley R. Kern, "Issues of competency in the aged," *Psychiatric Annals* 17, no. 5 (May 1987): 336–339.

[7] B. Myers and C. L. Barrett, "Competency issues in referrals to a consultation-liaison service," *Psychosomatics* 27, no. 11 (November 1986): 782–789, doi: 10.1016/S0033-3182(86)72605-4. PMID: 3797610.

[8] P. S. Appelbaum and T. Grisso, "Assessing patients' capacities to consent to treatment," *New England Journal of Medicine* 319, no. 25 (December 1988): 1635–1638, doi: 10.1056/NEJM198812223192504.

[9] Christopher Libby, Amanda Wojahn, Joseph R. Nicolini, and Gary Gillette, "Competency and capacity," The National Institutes of Health, accessed April 24, 2023, https://www.ncbi.nlm.nih.gov/books/NBK532862/.

[10] Raphael J. Leo, "Competency and the capacity to make treatment decisions: A primer for primary care physicians," *Primary Care Companion Journal of Clinical Psychiatry* 1, no. 5 (October 1999): 131–141, doi: 10.4088/pcc.v01n0501. PMID: 15014674; PMCID: PMC181079.

[11] P. S. Appelbaum and L. H. Roth, "Competency to consent to research: A psychiatric overview," *Archives of General Psychiatry* 39, no. 8 (August 1982): 951–958, doi: 10.1001/archpsyc.1982.04290080061009.

[12] Thomas Gilbert, Antoine Bosquet, Catherine Thomas-Antérion, Marc Bonnefoy, and Olivia Le Saux, "Assessing capacity to consent for research in cognitively impaired older patients," *Clinical Interventions in Aging* 12 (September 2017): 1553–1563, doi: 10.2147/CIA.S141905. PMID: 29026293; PMCID: PMC5627738.

Pausing for a moment, he then said, "I don't think the nation's quite ready, but I hope that somebody might get people to start thinking about this. . . . I believe that giving this option to individuals who have Alzheimer's is going to make their lives better as they live with the disease."

Until he expressed this opinion, I had not entirely appreciated why Dan was confiding to me the intimate details of his life. Yes, I've always been easy to talk to and curious about people's stories, which is part of why I gravitated to psychiatry. My medical background and previous books had made it apparent to Dan that I would be knowledgeable about neuropsychiatric clinical issues and sympathetic to those who wished to take control of their deaths. However, Dan was now being explicit that he had an agenda—which I soon learned John shared—and it involved encouraging people with dementias to demand more and better end-of-life options. If inclusion in official MAiD protocols was a stretch right now, then he and John wanted Americans to at least be more understanding of why folk with dementing illnesses might choose to arrange rational suicides on their own. The two men understood that our society's complex reaction to the concept of suicide has a lot to do with how the MAiD laws were formulated and why people with dementia have been effectively excluded.

Oregon's Death with Dignity Act explicitly states that ending one's life in accordance with the statute does not constitute suicide; actions taken in accord with the statute shall not for any purpose constitute suicide, assisted suicide, mercy killing, or homicide.[13] Furthermore, the Oregon Health Authority Center for Health Statistics recommends that physicians record the underlying terminal disease as being the cause of death (e.g., breast cancer, etc.). They are instructed to list the manner of death as being "natural."[14] But these provisions, which have been echoed in subsequent American assisted dying laws, have not stopped society from debating whether this practice is a means to abet suicide and whether it is acceptable and compassionate or immoral and monstrous.

In her 2016 book, legal scholar Susan Stefan began by asking a provocative question: Is suicide a public health scourge or an essential civil right?[15] She inquires: "Should it always be prevented, with state intervention if necessary, as

---

[13] Margaret P. Battin, Thaddeus M. Pope, and Lonny Shavelson, "Medical aid in dying: Ethical and legal issues," accessed August 13, 2023, https://www.uptodate.com/contents/medical-aid-in-dying-ethical-and-legal-issues?search=aid%20in%20dying&source=search_result&selectedTitle=2~150&usage_type=default&display_rank=2.

[14] "Oregon's Death with Dignity Act (DWDA): Frequently asked questions," Oregon Health Authority, accessed April 21, 2023, https://www.oregon.gov/oha/ph/providerpartnerresources/evaluationresearch/deathwithdignityact/pages/faqs.aspx#deathcert.

[15] Susan Stefan, *Rational Suicide, Irrational Laws: Examining Current Approaches to Suicide in Policy and Law* (New York: Oxford University Press, 2016), xv–xvi.

Justice Antonin Scalia and many mental health professionals believe? Is it a fundamental right that the state cannot interfere with, as the ACLU and Dr. Thomas Szasz have concluded?"[16] She argues that America's public, its policies, and laws—and for that matter, those of most other countries—"struggle in the murky middle" and are inconsistent and conflicted.

A. Alvarez wrote: "For suicide is, after all, the result of a choice. However impulsive the action and confused the motives, at the moment when a man finally decides to take his own life he achieves a certain temporary clarity . . . at least to this one decision which, by its very finality, is not wholly a failure."[17]

Alvarez and others have delved into the early background of suicide, and they cite a history replete with superstitious horror, vindictiveness, and degradation. .[18,19,20] They allude to how even in the enlightened Athens of Plato, as well as in the city-states of Thebes and Sparta, the bodies of people who killed themselves were routinely buried outside the municipality's boundaries after their "self-murdering" hands were cut off. In Medieval Europe, the corpses of commoners had a stake driven through the chest and were interred at the crossroads where passersby would walk on top of them. On other occasions, a stone was placed over the suicide's face to prevent his or her ghost from rising.[21] French and English nobles were demoted to the status of commoners immediately following suicide, and their property was confiscated by the crown. In England, the seizure of property went on until the 19th century, and an ineffective suicide could still result in imprisonment as late as 1961. According to Alvarez, as recently as 1969, a court in the Isle of Man sentenced a teenager to be birched for attempting suicide.

But nowadays most citizens of privileged nations recognize it doesn't make logical sense to criminalize such behavior, and, when cases appear before juries, the individuals who sit in judgment often ignore or choose to intentionally distort any existing criminal laws relating to suicide and assisted suicide.[22] In the United Kingdom and United States, suicide was finally stricken from the rolls as

---

[16] Thomas Szasz, *Suicide Prohibition: The Shame of Medicine* (Syracuse, NY: Syracuse University Press, 2011), 45.

[17] A. Alvarez, *The Savage God: A Study of Suicide* (New York: Random House, 1970).

[18] Margaret Pabst Battin, *The Ethics of Suicide: Historical Sources* (New York: Oxford University Press, 2015).

[19] Georges Minois, *A History of Suicide: Voluntary Death in Western Culture* (Baltimore, MD: Johns Hopkins University Press, 1999).

[20] Alvarez, *The Savage God*, 6, 45–72.

[21] Lewis M. Cohen, *No Good Deed: A Story of Medicine, Murder Accusations, and the Debate over How We Die* (New York: Harper Collins, 2010), 80–81.

[22] Alvarez, *The Savage God*, 14.

a statutory crime in the middle of the 20th century,[23] although some states still consider it to be a common law crime.[24]

Dr. Jack Kevorkian was tried on four separate occasions for assisting suicides, acquitted three times, and the judge declared a mistrial in the fourth case. He was only convicted during a fifth trial, which was convened after a *60 Minutes* broadcast showed him injecting Thomas Youk, who suffered from Lou Gehrig's disease (amyotrophic lateral sclerosis), with a dose of lethal drugs. At the trial, Dr. Kevorkian also refused to rely on his long-time and skilled attorney who had previously represented him.[25]

Suicide remains a crime in at least 20 countries, including Bangladesh, India, Malaysia, Pakistan, and Nigeria.[26] North Korea's law takes matters a step further by punishing family members of suicide victims.[27]

While one might think that Anglo-American psychiatrists uniformly believe that suicide is a product of mental illness and should be uniformly prohibited and/or aggressively treated, such is not necessarily the case. Admittedly, most psychiatrists subscribe to this position, but, upon further reflection, many would maintain that killing oneself can be right *or* wrong and is sometimes an element of one's inalienable personal liberty.[28] Medical professionals struggle like the rest of us for an answer to the questions: In a world without God, and when society no longer sees the taking of one's own life as a sin, what does suicide mean? How should we respond to those who choose to end life or those who help them?[29]

The aforementioned psychiatric iconoclast, Dr. Thomas Szasz (d. September 8, 2012), affirmed, "In principle, killing oneself is not different from other acts

[23] Lewis M. Cohen, *A Dignified Ending: Taking Control Over How We Die* (Lanham, MD: Rowman & Littlefield, 2019).

[24] Stefan, *Rational Suicide*, 18–19.

[25] Keith Schneider, "Dr. Jack Kevorkian dies at 83: A doctor who helped end lives," *The New York Times*, accessed January 12, 2022, https://www.nytimes.com/2011/06/04/us/04kevorkian.html.

[26] Sarah Johnson, "Suicide still treated as a crime in at least 20 countries, report finds," *The Guardian*, accessed September 23, 2022, https://www.theguardian.com/global-development/2021/sep/09/suicide-still-treated-as-a-in-at-least-20-countries-report-finds.

[27] Farhana H. Mehtab, Arif Mahmud, Riaduzzaman, Mahabub U. I. Alam Khan Emon, and Fariha Hossen, "Right to commit suicide in India: A comparative analysis with suggestion for the policymakers," *Cogent Social Sciences* 8, no. 1 (December 2022), doi: 10.1080/23311886.2021.2017574.

[28] Thomas Szasz, *Fatal Freedom: The Ethics and Politics of Suicide* (New York: Syracuse University Press, 1999; 2002), ix.

[29] Nina Power and Pierre d'Alancaisez, "In a world without God, what does suicide mean? When society no longer sees the taking of one's own life as a sin, it is unclear who should be responsible for attempting to prevent such deaths," *The Critic*, accessed August 14, 2023, https://thecritic.co.uk/issues/august-september-2023/in-a-world-without-god-what-does-suicide-mean/.

that have far-reaching irreversible consequences, such as begetting a child. The person who kills himself does so because he deems terminating his life preferable to continuing it. If we agree with his judgement, we call his suicide 'rational'; if we do not, we call it 'irrational.'"

Like many aid-in-dying proponents, Thomas Strouse, MD, Professor of Clinical Psychiatry and the Maddie Katz Endowed Chair in Palliative Care Research and Education at UCLA, is cautious about using the word "suicide." Dr. Strouse told me (October 29, 2022) that he supports "the autonomous rights of decisionally competent persons to contemplate and to complete rational self-delivery in the setting of life-limiting medical illness." He is an articulate advocate of state laws that outline how willing professionals can participate in supporting such patients' assertion of autonomy by providing legal lethal prescriptions that constitute MAiD. Dr. Strouse takes the position that palliative care clinicians who refuse to participate in MAiD and also don't facilitate access to a willing professional are demonstrating a "toxic form of patient abandonment."[30,31]

In a previous position statement, the American Association of Suicidology tried to further clarify these matters and wrote: "[The practice of physician aid in dying] is distinct from the behavior that has been traditionally and ordinarily described as 'suicide,' the tragic event our organization works so hard to prevent. Although there may be overlap between the two categories, legal physician-assisted deaths should not be considered suicide."[32] The Association's opinion concluded that suicide and physician aid in dying are "conceptually, medically, and legally different phenomena."

Susan Stefan, JD, has taken a nuanced position. She points out a lack of consensus among European countries regarding assisted suicide, and how some of these consider the exclusion of people with neuropsychiatric disabilities— like Dan—to be *illegal discrimination* unless the individuals have been declared incompetent.[33] But Professor Stefan opines: "One of the most important objections to physician-assisted suicide [is] that lethal medications are very rarely prescribed by a physician who has a long relationship with the patient. For the most part, medications are prescribed by a physician who strongly believes

---

[30] Thomas B. Strouse, "Oncology clinicians should understand end-of-life options including legal pathways to physician aid in dying," *Journal of Communication and Support in Oncology* 15, no. 1 (2017): 1–3.

[31] Thomas B. Strouse, "Editor's reply: Toxic abandonment and the case against physician participation in aid in dying," *Journal of Communication and Support in Oncology* 15, no. 2 (2017): 122–124.

[32] "AAS PAD statement approved October 30, 2017," American Association of Suicidology, accessed October 17, 2022, https://suicidology.org/wp-content/uploads/2019/07/AAS-PAD-Statement-Approved-10.30.17-ed-10-30-17.pdf.

[33] Susan Stefan, "A medical degree is not a license to prescribe death," *Psychiatric Times* 39, no. 12 (December 2022), accessed December 8, 2022.

in the concept of physician-assisted suicide. In my opinion, a medical degree and an agenda are not sufficient to license someone to prescribe death to another person."

She goes on to say: "I continue to feel that medicalizing an essentially personal and philosophical decision is a mistake. Suicide is not 'treatment,' and I resist categorizing it this way."[34]

This last statement is echoed by geriatrician and policy authority Dr. Joanne Lynn, who has long maintained that society's emphasis should be on the provision of *better* care for people who are very sick, disabled, or elderly. "We should resist medical aid in dying until we can offer a real choice of a well-supported, meaningful, and comfortable existence to people who would have chosen a medically assisted death," Dr. Lynn said. "There's currently no strong push for decency in long-term care. It's not a real choice if a person's alternative is living in misery or impoverishing the family."[35]

Psychiatrist and suicidologist Dr. J. Michael Bostwick has been my research collaborator. He takes exception to those who would challenge Dan and label his plan for death as being a suicide. He writes (January 15, 2023, email): "Dan proposes a course of action that is the antithesis of the desperate act of an individual unilaterally and often impulsively choosing to end an unbearable existence. Dan has carefully charted the course of his proposed exit. He has made no secret that he considers succumbing to the ravages of dementia to be a fate worse than death. He has discussed his intentions with his care providers and loved ones, gaining their assent or at least their understanding. He has enlisted their help in so far as they feel morally or legally able to provide it. Even if he can't rely on his state's assistance due to its blanket exclusion of those with dementia, regardless of whether they still retain capacity, he is neither alone nor depressed as he takes charge of his final destiny."

And Dr. Bostwick is correct that most *clinical suicides* are impulsive acts. According to a review article, among people who made near-lethal suicide attempts, 24% took less than 5 minutes between the decision to kill themselves and the actual attempt, while 70% took less than an hour.[36] This hardly describes Dan's situation.

Dan was also quick to underscore his repulsion at the idea of resorting to a *violent suicide* by using a gun or jumping from the roof of a building.[37] Such

[34] Stefan, *Rational Suicide*, 179–220.

[35] Jane E. Brody, "When patients choose to end their lives: For some, the decision to die is more complicated than a wish to reduce pain," *The New York Times*, accessed May 18, 2023, https://www.nytimes.com/2021/04/05/well/live/aid-in-dying.html.

[36] Seena Fazel and Bo Runeson, "Suicide," *New England Journal of Medicine* 382 (January 2020):266–274, doi: 10.1056/NEJMra1902944.

[37] Laurie Loisel, *On Their Own Terms: How One Woman's Choice to Die Helped Me Understand My Father's Suicide* (Amherst, MA: Levellers Press, 2019).

methods were anathema to him, although firearms are a common means of suicide among people with dementia.

Gun safety advocate Dr. Emmy Betz clarified that in at least one research investigation, 73% of suicide deaths in the context of dementia involved the use
of a firearm, in comparison with 50% of suicide deaths in people of all ages.[38]
In 2022, U.S. suicides hit an all-time high, and the largest increases were seen in
older adults, where deaths rose more than 8% in people 65 and older.[39] White
men, in particular, have very high rates, according to the U.S. Centers for Disease
Control (CDC).[40] Roughly half of adults aged 65 years or older have a gun in
the home,[41] and Dr. Betz has been trying to encourage the limitation of firearm
access for people with cognitive impairments. Elderly men who commit suicide
using a firearm are typically white, married veterans who have physical health
problems, reside in rural areas, and are *less* likely to have made previous suicide
attempts.[42] In a recent study of older adults, three-fourths of suicide decedents
did *not* inform others of their intent to commit suicide. This study also found
that almost 82% of males who killed themselves with a firearm were *not* known
to have a mental illness.[43]

Dr. Betz's campaign seems logical, especially when viewed through the lens of
a recent study of 2.7 million older adults in the United States diagnosed with dementia by Dr. Timothy Schmutte and associates from Yale University School of
Medicine.[44] He wrote me (December 21, 2022, email) that 63% of these suicide

[38] Emmy Betz, "Dr. Emmy Betz: Exploring the ties between firearms and suicide," Everytown
Research & Policy, accessed September 23, 2022, https://everytownresearch.org/dr-emmy-betz-
exploring-the-ties-between-firearms-and-suicide/.

[39] Mike Stobbe, "U.S. suicides hit an all-time high last year," The Associated Press, accessed
August 13, 2023, https://apnews.com/article/suicides-record-2022-guns-48511d74deb24d933
e66cec1b6f2d545.

[40] "Suicide data and statistics," Centers for Disease Control and Prevention, accessed August 13,
2023, https://www.cdc.gov/suicide/suicide-data-statistics.html.

[41] Kim Parker, Juliana Menasce Horowitz, Ruth Igielnik, J. Baxter Oliphat, and Anna Brown,
"America's complex relationship with guns: An in-depth look at the attitudes and experiences of
U.S. adults," Pew Research Center, accessed December 21, 2022, https://www.pewresearch.org/soc
ial-trends/2017/06/22/americas-complex-relationship-with-guns/.

[42] U.S. Department of Health and Human Services, Office of the Surgeon General, "2012 national strategy for suicide prevention: Goals and objectives for action: A report of the US Surgeon
General and of the National Action Alliance for Suicide Prevention," accessed November 17, 2020,
https://www.ncbi.nlm.nih.gov/books/NBK109917/.

[43] Timothy J. Schmutte and Samuel T. Wilkinson, "Suicide in older adults with and without known
mental illness: Results from the National Violent Death Reporting System, 2003–2016," *American
Journal of Preventive Medicine* 58, no. 4 (April 2020): 584–590., doi: 10.1016/j.amepre.2019.11.001.

[44] Timothy Schmutte, Mark Olfson, Donovan T. Maust, Ming Xie, and Steven Marcus, "Suicide
risk in first year after dementia diagnosis in older adults," *Alzheimers & Dementia* 18, no. 2 (February
2022): 262–271, doi: 10.1002/alz.12390.

deaths involved the use of firearms. The suicide rates in the first year following a dementia diagnosis were 53% higher than the already elevated suicide rate in the general geriatric population. Even larger increases in risk were observed for certain demographic groups (e.g., females, persons of color, and adults aged 65–74 years), which ranged from 104% to 240% higher. Other authorities have pointed out that access to firearms may pose a dual danger for both the elderly with dementing disorders and their family members.[45]

In a call for action, Drs. Price and Khubchandani concluded that the handguns used by the elderly for suicides are usually purchased decades earlier, and the most effective interventions ought to involve strengthening state firearm laws to remove them from the homes, as well as efforts to improve mental healthcare.[46] Experts suggest that a diagnosis of cognitive impairment does not necessarily preclude safe gun ownership, but doctors aren't trained to initiate or discuss these preventable tragedies by effectively dealing with families.[47]

Among the most heartrending stories that I have followed is that of Pam and Stephen Kruspe.[48,49] Mrs. Kruspe had been committed to a Florida assisted living facility because of early-onset Alzheimer's disease, when she asked her husband, a retired Marine, to shoot her. Apparently after considerable soul-searching, he acquiesced and then immediately turned himself in to law enforcement. After confessing, Mr. Kruspe was promptly arrested and charged with premeditated first-degree murder. He spent much of the following 6 years awaiting a trial delayed by clogged courts and COVID-19. During that time, he faced a potential sentence of life in prison. According to Kruspe's attorney, "He wants his story told. He wants a jury to know not just what he did—but why."

Kruspe described to the police how, "For months, she had been telling me . . . the anguish she was going through . . . just unbelievable . . . like a horror story. . . . She said, 'I don't want to be here. I want to die. I want you to kill me.' . . . It went on and on. I couldn't take it anymore."

[45] Brian Mertens and Susan B. Sorenson, "Current considerations about the elderly and firearms," *American Journal of Public Health* 102, no. 3 (March 2012): 396–400, doi: 10.2105/AJPH.2011.300404.

[46] James H. Price and Jagdish Khubchandani, "Firearm suicides in the elderly: A narrative review and call for action," *Journal of Community Health* 46, no. 5 (October 2021): 1050–1058, doi: 10.1007/s10900-021-00964-7. Epub 2021 Feb 5. PMID: 33547617; PMCID: PMC7864138.

[47] Alan Drummond, "It's time to talk about dementia, firearms and suicide," *Ottawa Citizen*, accessed March 23, 2023, https://ottawacitizen.com/health/men/drummond-its-time-to-talk-about-dementia-firearms-and-suicide.

[48] Cohen, *A Dignified Ending*, 15–26, 53–61.

[49] Lane DeGregory, "After a Florida father shoots his wife, a family fractures," *Tampa Bay Times*, accessed September 23, 2022, https://www.tampabay.com/news/2022/01/08/after-a-florida-father-shoots-his-wife-a-family-fractures/.

But that account doesn't satisfy everyone.

At a hearing, Kruspe's daughter angrily read from a letter she wrote that argued why her father should remain in jail. "To have and to hold, for better or for worse, in sickness and in health is not demonstrated," she said, "by a .45 to the chest."

In March of 2023, Kruspe pleaded guilty to manslaughter by assisted suicide.[50] In September, he received a sentence of 20 years. According to the *Tampa Bay Times*, with credit for time served, Kruspe will be 83 when he can walk free.[51]

But he knows that he will never be free.

[50] Hannah Phillips, "Mercy or murder? Marine vet who assisted ailing wife's suicide pleads guilty to manslaughter," *Palm Beach Post*, accessed April 3, 2023, https://www.palmbeachpost.com/story/news/crime/2023/03/28/marine-vet-pleads-guilty-to-manslaughter-assisting-wifes-suicide/69855773007/.

[51] Lane DeGregory, "For a Florida Marine who killed his wife, a life sentence or leniency?," *Tampa Bay Times*, accessed February 7, 2024, https://www.tampabay.com/news/crime/2023/09/15/husband-shot-wife-assisted-suicide-sentence/

Around the same time Dan reflexively dismissed the idea of relying on a weapon or other violent means to end his life, he considered and then rejected the practice of voluntarily stopping eating and drinking (VSED). He did not wish to engage in "a long-drawn-out process or a bedside vigil." He didn't want to "go into a coma before death," and he knew that fasting could take up to a month, which was "just putting too much pressure on people."

Dan further explained, "I want my loved ones to know that I'm going to be gone by this specific date. I want to have certainty for them . . . VSED just sounds like an unnecessary way to die when you can do it safely, cleanly, and all at once with medications." A "pharmaceutical overdose" made more sense to him.

Dan initially considered ending his life in the fall of 2020, but he then changed his mind and shifted to either December 17 or 31. However, Dan was saddened at the thought of the extended Winter family recalling the anniversary of his death during future holiday seasons.

He wanted to openly talk about the suicide plan but couldn't figure out whether there was an established etiquette covering how to inform people. When Dan originally tried broaching the subject, some of his friends thought he was joking and nervously laughed at his remarks. When this occurred, he felt disappointed with their lack of empathy. Afterward, when his mood darkened, he thought, *Wait a minute, how narcissistic are you to believe that they're going to even give a fuck?*

But Dan was serious about his intentions, and, when we first spoke, he was at the tail end of assembling "a lethal cocktail of medications." A key component was the tricyclic antidepressant amitriptyline hydrochloride, often sold under the brand name Elavil, which is used to treat major depressive disorder and a variety of pain syndromes. Dan had done his reading and received guidance from several right-to-die activists.[1] He planned on combining a massive dose, along with an antinausea pill, alcohol, and antianxiety medication.

---

[1] Boudewijn Chabot, *Dignified Dying: Guide to Humane Self-Chosen Death* (Amsterdam: Foundation Dignified Dying, 2006), 47–48.

The 17th-century poet John Donne wrote, "Whensoever my affliction assails me, methinks I have the keys of my prison in mine own hand, and no remedy presents itself so soon to my heart, as mine own sword."[2] To many people, like Dan, that meant they should have the right to take their lives. However, countless thousands have found out the hard way that there are a myriad of different ways to *fail* at achieving this goal, including falsely assuming that large amounts of morphine, benzodiazepines, or acetaminophen are always effective—they are not.

More than a quarter-century ago, Derek Humphry, founder of the Hemlock Society, and Dr. Lonny Shavelson, an inspirational leader of American medical aid in dying, spoke at a public forum in front of more than 150 predominantly gay men who were suffering from AIDS in San Francisco. The subject was botched suicide attempts and the potential legal consequences involving loved ones.

Humphry explained that too many people who wished to die "were taking the wrong medication at the wrong times and having bad outcomes. [These] included things like partial overdoses, where people would fall asleep for 2 days from an overdose of morphine that did not result in death but resulted in brain damage. And they'd wake up 2 days later, sicker than they started and with even more suffering."[3]

Humphry and Dr. Shavelson cautioned against using kitchen chemicals and random pills from the medicine cabinet that were more likely to result in the would-be-suicide having his or her stomach pumped in a hospital emergency room. The two men discouraged their audience from relying on automobile exhaust asphyxiation, which became even less feasible following the institution of pollution controls and catalytic converters. They warned against using violent suicide methods, like hanging or self-inflicted gunshot wounds, which they pointed out are traumatizing to families, passersby, and first responders.

Humphry concluded: "Mix in circles that care about these things and you'll pick up information about people who are courageous and leave nothing to chance. Do not skimp on the details. A well-planned self-deliverance almost always works."[4]

For many years in the United States, the fast-acting barbiturates secobarbital and pentobarbital had been the preferred drugs of choice for legal executions,

[2] John Donne, "Biathanatos (1608)," LibQuotes, accessed June 8, 2023, https://libquotes.com/john-donne/quote/lbb2w8i.

[3] JoAnn Marr, "How one viral video helped make aid-in-dying possible in California," Crosscurrents, accessed September 23, 2022, https://www.kalw.org/show/crosscurrents/2017-02-02/how-one-viral-video-helped-make-aid-in-dying-possible-in-california.

[4] Jane Gross, "At AIDS epicenter, seeking swift, sure death," *New York Times*, accessed June 7, 2023, https://www.nytimes.com/1993/06/20/us/at-aids-epicenter-seeking-swift-sure-death.html.

and these have likewise been employed under physician aid-in-dying laws or used in rational suicides—like that of Sandra Bem. In the Netherlands, these medications continue to be relied upon for assisted dying; however, the barbiturates are respiratory suppressants—meaning, they stop or slow the rate of breathing. While they rapidly place *most* people into a coma and can result in death approximately 25 minutes after ingestion, *some* individuals linger for up to 4 days after receiving these overdoses. The barbiturates have now also become difficult to reliably obtain because counterfeit drugs are all too common.

When physicians in Oregon and Washington State began using secobarbital routinely in those communities' death-with-dignity protocols, they came to further appreciate the medication's shortcomings. Their observations led a few doctors from Washington to explore the use of alternative drugs, such as digitalis and propranolol, which trigger death by causing the heart to stop beating.

More recently, a group of medical providers, the American Clinicians Academy on Medical Aid in Dying, headed up by Dr. Shavelson, have been pooling their experience with various combinations of medications to arrive at recommendations that are more effective, rapid, and less likely to result in side effects.[5] They have decided that ideally the components need to be widely available for common medical conditions, relatively inexpensive, and painless to ingest. The practitioners are acquiring data on the mean time to death after administration, the presence of complications, maximum time to death, and other variables.

The group's members rely on compounding pharmacies to assemble the fatal draughts with powder and liquid ingredients. Compounding pharmacies are scattered throughout the United States, and they make drugs prescribed by doctors for specific patients who have needs that cannot be met with available medications.[6] An example would be a young child who requires a small, liquid dose of a drug that is commercially made only in adult-dosage tablets.

DDMAPh is currently the Academy's preferred, lethal combination drug of choice, and it includes digitalis, diazepam, morphine, amitriptyline, and phenobarbital. In several email exchanges with Dr. Shavelson (October 11, 2022), he explained how analysis of data from 175 patients ound that 85% of the sample died within 2 hours or less. About 3% of individuals survived for between 5 and 10 hours. The sample has since increased to more than 1,000 patients (August 15, 2023) as clinicians keep reporting results to the Academy.

[5] American Clinicians Academy on Medical Aid in Dying, accessed September 23, 2022, https://www.acamaid.org/.

[6] "Compounding and the FDA: Questions and answers," U.S. Food & Drug Administration, accessed June 7, 2023, https://www.fda.gov/drugs/human-drug-compounding/compounding-and-fda-questions-and-answers.

Because Dan was ineligible for medical aid in dying, he could not obtain DDMAPh. Instead, he intended to assemble his own cocktail from separate prescriptions of different medications. I was never sure about who was advising Dan regarding the type, amount, and sequence for ingesting the mixture of pharmaceuticals, but I hoped for his sake that he was getting trustworthy guidance. Since drugs are developed to *cure* disorders or *manage* symptoms—and their purpose is *not* to help people to die—most doctors lack basic knowledge regarding how one might use medications to intentionally cause death. Many pills also contain a substantial amount of inert "fillers," so trying to exactly duplicate a compound like DDMAPh with individual prescriptions is unwieldy and impractical.

Dan sat down with John and a physician; the latter agreed to hear the basics of his plan to overdose before the Alzheimer's symptoms became intolerable. "She got it," Dan explained. "She did not try to talk me out of it, and she wrote the requested script for the amitriptyline with three or four additional refills."

He paused and said, "So, just to summarize, I told a complete stranger who's a medical professional that I was going to kill myself, and she looked and acted supportive."

"But then," Dan said with astonishment, "I asked her for a Xanax script to help with my anxiety. And she said—"

Interrupting him, I exclaimed, "I can guess!" Then restraining myself, I muttered an apologetic, "Sorry, go on."

"She said, 'Xanax? No, that's too habit forming.' " Dan paused for a second and sounded incredulous when he continued, "So, I'm looking at the prescription in my hand with four refills of 60 tablets of 100 milligrams each of Elavil. . . . "

"That she's just given you."

"After I told her in front of my husband that I am going to kill myself."

Dan and I paused for a moment, and then we agreed it was an absurd situation even if it was understandable.[7]

The two of us gingerly talked about the process that led him to this drug combination, and I inquired, "Do you want to tell me who provided the information?"

"Well," he said, "I'll give you a tiny bit of background. I started knowing that the method I wanted to utilize would result in a peaceful, nonviolent death. I bought updated copies of *Final Exit* and *The Peaceful Pill* [the books read by Sandy Bem before her suicide]. The barbiturate [Nembutal] that Sandy

[7] C. Jewett and E. Gabler, "Opioid settlement hinders patients' access to a wide array of drugs," *The New York Times*, March 13, 2023, accessed March 13, 2023, https://www.nytimes.com/2023/03/13/us/drug-limits-adhd-depression.html?campaign_id=2&emc=edit_th_20230313&instance_id=87459&nl=todaysheadlines&regi_id=63340269&segment_id=127631&user_id=895343099129dcd1f95fa65a5a136796.

relied upon is impossible to find in the United States, and I was not going to go to Mexico. It made me uncomfortable to contemplate ordering such a thing through the mail."

He went on, "I'd gotten as far with the Final Exit Network (FEN) [an American aid-in-dying nonprofit organization largely composed of volunteers who educate and emotionally support people suffering from physical illnesses to take their lives] to have been assigned a. . . . Oh, what do they call it?"

" 'An 'exit guide?' " I ventured.

"A guide? Right." he continued. "And that guide was a delightful, helpful, and thoughtful woman. But I wasn't comfortable being in the FEN community. There was just a . . . I don't know . . . " He stumbled over his words for a while and then said, "I certainly believe in what they do."

FEN works with people who either don't live in states having medical aid in dying laws or who don't meet the eligibility criteria—like Dan. Guides undergo formal training and quietly operate in the shadows. The organization specifically has an initiative in which they offer to provide legal representation to people with dementia whose advance directives—and FEN has designed a good one—are being ignored. An example would be a nursing home that continues to push spoon feeding when the living will and healthcare proxy have stated that the individual's wish is to the contrary.

Rob Rivas, JD, the attorney for FEN, wrote me (June 14, 2023, email): "I'm not sure it's fair to say FEN 'operates in the shadows.' Everything FEN does is on its website and is publicized in every way possible. This is contrary to the notion that FEN operates in the shadows. Still, I see references like this all the time. They are fueled by the confidentiality FEN imposes on direct relations with recipients of Exit Guide services. Obviously, the volunteers can't let the family members know anything about a planned exit or the family members might interfere. Measures are taken to ensure the family members know about the exit and are okay with it, or at least won't obstruct. Measures are taken to actually involve the closest family members whenever possible.

" 'Secrecy,' if that's what to call it, also requires that healthcare providers and law enforcement don't find out because the person who exits doesn't want this to come out after the exit. We have to respect that. There's always the possibility that a local news medium would think it's newsworthy if a person's death was an 'assisted suicide' connected to the 'shadowy' FEN. We wouldn't mind that other than the unconscionable breach of the decedent's confidentiality.

"Many volunteers talk about how great it would be if clients would sometimes come out and let FEN's involvement be publicly known after the exit. But we can't promote or even suggest a person make this decision because of the conflict of interest involved, i.e., the exiting person would feel pressured to cooperate in publicizing FEN's volunteer services. We don't mention the idea of posthumously going public, and the subject would be considered only in the vanishingly rare instance of someone saying they would like to publicize their death to promote the public policy issue."

Dan continued stammering to me about why FEN wasn't a suitable fit, and he said, "For some reason . . . I can't put my finger on it . . . but whatever it is, it wasn't for me."

I did not pursue this line of questioning with him but suspect that his reticence may have had mostly to do with FEN's preferred reliance on the use of nitrogen gas to hasten death, rather than recommending the use of oral medication overdoses. An inert gas, like nitrogen, is considered to be fast, efficient, and doesn't result in any sensation of asphyxiation because it shuts down the brain's breathing center. However, many people consider it esthetically displeasing or undignified to strap a bag over one's head (ordinarily used to cook turkeys) that is attached by a tube to a gas cannister. Furthermore, if one does not wish for the authorities to know that you've carried out the "exit," "self-deliverance," or "chosen death"—alternative terms used frequently within the right-to-die community—then another person needs to afterward remove and dispose of the apparatus. On the other hand, I have been told that consciousness is lost after just a couple of breaths of nitrogen, and that death ensues within a few minutes.

Upon reading this paragraph, the bioethicist David N. Hoffman wrote to me (email June 24, 2023): "There are, of course, no shortage of methods for any individual ending their life. Whether the act is considered legally or morally permissible or justifiable, is largely irrelevant when somebody has decided that the burdens of living outweigh the benefits. What most patients I have encountered want, and what our society should make possible, is a process for ending one's life that is *safe, certain,* and *painless.* If objectors assert that by making such an ending of life possible we are encouraging suicide, I would challenge that individual's right to create obstacles to a *safe, certain,* and *painless* death as a means of manipulating the patient's opportunities."

Dan summed up our conversation about FEN by saying, "I instead connected with a couple of local activists, who told me more about amitriptyline."

13

The next time we spoke Dan sounded distraught, and he remarked, "My symptoms are 'ramping up.'" He went on to say: "My cognitive performance after four o'clock in the afternoon is not good compared to ten o'clock in the morning. I can still cook though, and that's a respite. If I make mistakes and put in a cup of baking powder when it should be a cup of sugar—that'll sure ruin a dish. But I continue to enjoy cooking and just made a hell of a chocolate mocha cake."

Our interview felt disjointed. I could feel my face locking into a frozen smile, something I do when things get awkward and uncomfortable. In retrospect, I didn't want to hear about how the disease was progressing. Rather than elicit more about his suffering, I asked, "What else are you enjoying?"

"I delight in the time I have in the morning," he said. "I get up several hours before John does. The dog wakes me up, which is fine. My early mornings by myself are a luxury. I read the paper. I have two newspapers—the one that's delivered and an online version."

Dan continued, "I'll read some news stories a couple of times if there's something that strikes me—like a piece about Melania Trump's new dress—because I can't really get it all done in one pass. That's frustrating but I'm still curious. I'm also enjoying every minute spent with John. He's retired, too. John's taken up painting again, and he has gotten represented by arguably the best gallery in town."

"Wow," I said.

"Yeah, it's really cool. I've also resigned from the ACLU national and state boards. . . . I know what's going to happen with this disease, and I really want to experience the quality of life that's left. I realize that being around my children is more important than anything. Being around their mother is vital. . . . Being around my siblings and my nieces and nephews. . . . All told, there's a group of about 17 men and women in my life, and I don't know what I would do without them."

I was momentarily incredulous when I thought about having such an enormous inner circle of beloveds.

John told me afterward, "Dan's such a smart, quick, curious man. He is remarkably well-read and was deeply engaged in Kansas City life. The first thing he did when he came here was to try and find ways to become involved in the civic culture of Portland. Now he has chosen to let go of those engagements. There's real emotional pain in not being able to be a part of the ACLU, which has been such a big piece of his identity for so many years."

"In addition," John said, "he had gotten involved with a group that's putting artwork in the organization that takes care of houseless and unhoused people in Portland, and while at first the idea sounded frivolous, it has turned out to be really meaningful to their clients. Volunteers, like Dan, express validation they haven't felt in a long time—that they are human enough to have artwork to look at and talk about. The nonprofit's staff can't get over what it is like to overhear their clients in the waiting room chatting about the meaning of this or that piece of art. It seems to take them completely out of a world that is otherwise primarily about suffering. It means a lot to Dan that there's now something like 1,000 pieces of original art in this collection, most of which are by Pacific Northwest artists."

"Am I safe in saying that he is no longer capable of participating in the organization or that kind of activity?" I asked.

"Yeah. Nothing he feels is meaningful. He's had to pull back from the activities that gave his life importance and pleasure. It's a genuine loss of his complex self."

*****

Dan further described to me the so-called rough sleepers—the homeless—in the Chinatown neighborhood where he resided.[1] He said, "There are a lot of social service agencies around. It's emotionally challenging to live among a population of folk who don't have a place to live. It grinds at me. Lately, their most common recreational activity seems to be dumping the contents of trash cans into the streets. When I look at the garbage strewn about, I shift from feeling despair, to feeling cranky, to feeling guilty."

"You were outside this morning and found your trash can overturned?" I asked.

"Oh, that's a daily thing," he replied. "The dumpsters from nearby businesses are always at least partially emptied. Three blocks away there's a park where I walk my dog, and every morning it seems like the cans have just been overturned.

[1] Tracy Kidder, *Rough Sleepers: Dr. Jim O'Connell's Urgent Mission to Bring Healing to Homeless People* (New York: Random House, 2023).

And then you realize they are overturned for understandable reasons: people are trying to find things that can be useful to them, like food. Or maybe it's just one way to show the world that they've got some control—because, frankly, they have no control over their lives. It's such an intractable tragedy.

"Ever since I got here, I've volunteered at an organization which offers jobs and training and medical care for those who don't have homes," said Dan. "I have regular contact with individuals inside the administration building who are trying to get services. But living amidst them and stepping over people to get to my condo doorway takes a little bite out of me every time. I've got all this privilege and I try to share it, but . . . there are limitations to what I can do."

"And you've been living in the Chinatown section of the city for how long now?" I inquired.

"We moved here last August. We had been living in a house that John and I built in a leafy inner-city neighborhood called Laurelhurst, which is just like it sounds. But it was just a bit slow for us. Plus, we wanted, considering my condition, to sell it and make our lives a little simpler. I gave up my driver's license when we moved here. I'm now adept at public transportation and ride my bicycle and walk when I can. And it's very, very convenient, as everything we need is down here. Everything! But also, the social problems that are inherent to this neighborhood."

*****

From the beginning, I decided that, given the dementia, it made the most sense for me to conduct separate interviews with Dan and John. This gave both men the opportunity to speak from their individual perspectives, and it offered me a chance to sometimes crosscheck Dan's statements. Since each of them was agreeable, we decided to conduct our interviews every couple of weeks.

Within the first minutes of our initial interview, John had told me, "to expect tears" on his part, and that I shouldn't worry. "It may be genetic," he joked—or maybe he was being serious. Either way, there were plenty of reasons in his life for him to be emotional, and, during our subsequent conversations, he certainly did a fair amount of crying.

The thing about John is that we instantly felt an intense connection. This was especially evident to me when he touchingly described the beginning of his relationship with Dan. He said, "Being 60 years old and Dan being 8 years younger than me, we'd both been around the block, and it wasn't like first love. There was a lot of the bullshit that just melted away. From very early on, we were able to be really safe with each other emotionally. I think he would say the same thing. I certainly felt it. Our experiences in life up to that point were enormously different. His family was Republican and deeply involved in Kansas politics, and they led lives that were cushioned by wealth and keenly tied to cultural expectations.

"Whereas I came from an entirely different kind of family," John continued, "and because I knew about my sexuality so much earlier, it framed my whole life in a way that sexuality did not frame Dan's. And so, he was from the beginning very curious about the differences in our lives. And I was curious about his. How had this man ended up being somebody that I immediately and deeply loved?

"Dan's avenue to the insights about himself was through his addiction and recovery with which I had no experience. While I had friends whose lives were saved by Alcoholics Anonymous, they didn't necessarily talk to me about their alcoholism. Dan was entirely forthcoming about that subject, and I was impressed by his willingness to look closely at who he was. I was genuinely moved by that quality.

"It took a little bit of time for him to open up about his sexual abuse. We were a committed couple when he relinquished trying to contain that shame. But I learned a lot from him. I did not know the extent of my ignorance . . . about how men groom the children they're going to abuse, or about the lifelong repercussions of rape."

John explained that "Dan's been consistent in his desire to end his own life from the very beginning of this disease. . . . His attitude has never varied, and he has never wavered during each conversation we've had on the subject. He's never had to convince me, since that would be my choice if I were in Dan's position."

John took a couple of deep breaths and said, "When Dan walked out of the neuropsychological testing sessions, it was his stated desire to *not* live out his life and have dementia be the ultimate cause of his death."

John took a shuddering breath and continued, "I instantly recognized that life was transformed forever. There was real difficulty in the future because of Dan's diagnosis. All that mattered was today . . . all that mattered was now. We both had a desire to *not* live in the future, to *not* catastrophize. Which is *not* to say that we avoided the future. However, we both independently appreciated the value of living in the moment."

He went on, "What followed was a period of transition, a continual and evolving recognition of the changes in Dan's health."

I remained silent.

"We just dealt with issues as they came up."

"Meaning?"

"He didn't always tell me immediately when there was a change . . . when something happened. The first time he had an auditory hallucination, he waited a couple of weeks to tell me. He waited until he was fully adjusted and more aware. I'm not sure 'adjusted' is the right word. He needed to know whether these alterations were progressing or continuing to happen before eventually telling me about them."

"Has Dan explicitly requested you to participate in ending his life?"

"No, he has never asked me to decide how he was going to do it or to help him get the drugs that are his choice of method. I'm not even privy right now as to whether he has finished collecting them. I don't ask."

"Why?"

"This is out of his desire to protect me from having any responsibility for the death."

"You're alluding to the potential legal and criminal ramifications?"

"Yup."

"Is he trying to protect you from the psychological impact of actively being involved in those decisions?

"Yeah, that, too. He doesn't want to put anyone else in the position of responsibility—whether it's his ex-wife, nieces and nephews, or his kids. He's been very careful and thoughtful about not having us become a part of that process."

John inhaled deeply and said, "A date has not been set, but it will probably take place by the end of this year. He's had long plateaus, and if there are no significant changes between now and the end of the year, he may choose to hold off. It's hard to project, but he is experiencing a lot of frustration."

"Over what?"

"When you list the specific things, they sound like no big deal. But using the phone is becoming more difficult. Using the remote control for the TV has become all but impossible. So, during the course of the day, he is unable to do things that he's been accustomed to doing. There's a roadblock just around every corner. Recently, reading has become more difficult. He can spend 10 minutes looking at two paragraphs of an article in *The Times* each morning. I don't know how much he's retaining and learning. He'll occasionally buy a book, but he hasn't finished one in quite some time. The pleasure or ability just isn't there anymore."

"The bottom line?"

"All that really matters is for me to support him through this," John replied.

14

Dan's situation was hardly taking place in a vacuum. In June 2020, when we spoke next, the COVID pandemic had erupted and was taking its toll. One of Dan and John's friends died from the virus, and the unexpected event hit them both hard.

This was combined with the killing of George Floyd, the leadup to the presidential election, and the City of Portland becoming convulsed by civil unrest and nightly protests. Antifa and the militias came out in force, and tumultuous demonstrations against police brutality and racism were punctuated by mayhem and looting. The sounds of chanting protestors and windows breaking echoed throughout downtown.

The riots that began to define Portland expanded to include many other causes, including a desire by some to defund the police. The Portland City Council voted to cut $15 million from the police budget, while activists demanded cuts of $50 million. The Council would later reverse course after an increase in shootings and murders. An 8 PM curfew in the city was adopted and then abandoned. The Portland Police Bureau Chief stepped down amid angry criticism that the department wasn't sufficiently diverse. A judge granted a temporary restraining order limiting law enforcement's use of tear gas and other crowd control munitions, while a reliance on clandestine FBI surveillance teams and militarized federal agents assigned to protect federal buildings stirred up concerns about government overreach.

John observed, "We were standing on our terrace one night and watched a couple of groups of eight to ten men dressed in black with hoodies—obviously out to intimidate people—approaching each other from different parts of the block and coming to an intersection in the street and then dispersing in several different directions. If I'd seen it on stage or in a film, it would have been a fascinating bit of choreography. But I'm deeply unsettled by the coordination of the radicals—it's hard to know whether it's radicals from the left or radicals from the right. Either way, right now, I'm kind of raw."

John's words reminded me about a newspaper article describing a New York City blackout, which began, "The looters scattered, roachlike, in the full morning sunlight, then stopped to watch brazenly."[1] The journalist then went on to say, "The darkness this time had a feral texture to it that seemed slow in dawning on the quieter parts of the city."

Dan added to this picture of municipal chaos by telling me how one of his regular 20-mile bike rides was interrupted by the appearance of "ten screaming cop cars barreling toward a small demonstration." Impulsively deciding to join the protestors, he chanted slogans with them for a few minutes before realizing that they were greatly outnumbered by the police and at any moment risked being arrested. Upon returning to the sanctuary of his apartment, Dan concluded, "It was all pretty visceral."

That night the sounds of helicopters with searchlights passing by overhead, police flash grenades exploding, street brawling, and extremists breaking into stores all combined to interfere with the two overtired men being able to fall asleep. They lay in bed and held each other, and it seemed as if they had been written into the script of a dystopian war film.

Meanwhile, Dan was preoccupied with his wish to "have a quiet death and avoid going through all the stages of this disease." He said, "I can see why, having decided to end my own life, I am not being secretive about it. I don't enjoy being preachy, but when I have an opportunity to talk then I'm pretty transparent about my intentions and my decisions."

"What drives you to speak?" I asked.

"I fear that there are people with dementias who don't feel they have the option to end their lives for religious reasons, family reasons, and other social pressures."

Dan was also troubled that the pills he planned on using might prove ineffective and he'd end up "a vegetable."

"It would be painfully ironic," I exclaimed.

Agreeing, Dan observed, "Alzheimer's is one long goodbye."[2]

Meanwhile, it was evident to me that John was anticipating and preparing. He observed how, "Dan always gets up before me. One morning, I came into the living room where he was sitting, and he had a certain look on his face. I told him, 'I imagine that expression on your face is what I'll see when you tell me it's

---

[1] Francis X, Clines, "About New York," *The New York Times*, accessed January 12, 2022, https://www.nytimes.com/1977/07/15/archives/about-new-york-down-these-mean-streets.html.

[2] "The long goodbye: Grieving someone with Alzheimer's," Journey to Joy Counseling, accessed August 23, 2023, https://www.journeytojoycounseling.com/2019/01/09/the-long-goodbye-grieving-someone-with-alzheimers/#:~:text=The%20reason%20Alzheimer's%20is%20referred,their%20life%20would%20look%20like

time.'" Pausing for a moment, John said, "Lew, that day is going to be horrible. There's no way out of this without it being horrible. But Dan is making it easier for the two of us by adamantly insisting that he is going to live his life out to the final minute."

John continued, "It goes back to what I was commenting on before: if you just look at him, if you just listen to him, it doesn't seem like what Dan is going through is such a big deal. But from the inside, he's experiencing the loss of himself all the time, and certainly, if he asks anything of me, I will do it."

*****

"Dan," I said. "Would you tell me more about your father's death? Were you present?"

"Most of the family assembled when we knew that he was finally at the end," Dan replied. "My older brother and I decided to stay with him while everybody else went to get showered and refreshed. The Kentucky Derby was playing on the television in his room."

Watching the horserace was an annual Winter event, mainly because Dan's grandfather had owned a thoroughbred. On this occasion, a close family friend, who happened to be a hospice nurse, sat down with them. Dan explained, "My dad was lying there in a coma. I glanced his way and noticed something was going on with his breathing. I asked her, 'What's happening here?'"

Dan swallowed, waited a second, and then said, "She walked over and took his pulse. Before she lay his hand down, our friend turned to us and softly said, 'He just passed away.'"

"My brother and I looked at each other, and strangely, we both had the same thought, *He would've been terribly depressed that he didn't get to finish watching the Derby.*

Dan continued, "But his wife, sister, my two brothers and I were all relieved. It wasn't that we weren't mourning him." Echoing his earlier statement, Dan said, "It's that Alzheimer's is a lengthy mourn. So, there wasn't an outpouring of grief."

He paused for a moment to collect his thoughts, and Dan then quietly reflected, "Wint Winter was a real character. A lot can be said about my dad—not all of it positive—but he was one of the most interesting people you'll ever encounter, and he really had a fantastic life. We celebrated that spirit when he was well; we weren't sorry when he died and his ordeal was over."

"I'm curious," I asked, "how do you imagine your own death?"

"I don't know," he said. "I know the method, and the cold hard facts are that it will involve amitriptyline as the delivery system. John and I talked last night. I told him that I wanted him to be there. I would love for each of my kids and their mother to be present a couple of days before, but it would not be a command performance. I want to respect each of them. I don't want to give the people I love the idea that I need them to be there when that relationship ends.

"It would be best," he said, "if the kids say their goodbyes before I take the medicine, so they can be out of the house. I'm not worried about the cops coming in to arrest them, or a wacky medical examiner or zealous prosecutor trying to incriminate my children. But I think that it would be best if there's evidence that everybody was gone ... this has to be done by me and me alone."

He went on, "At first, I had an idea that I was going to throw a party and let everybody know the date was sometime in the next 2 weeks. However, I realized the impracticality of such an approach. But I wish I could spend time now with friends and family outside of Portland."

Dan finished by saying, "I'm *not* worried about dying alone and feeling lonely, because John is going to be with me. I'm awfully fortunate to be with somebody who loves me, like he does."

Fortunate? *Fortunate*? Not exactly the word that I would have chosen. But the more I replayed our conversations, the more it seemed right.

*****

In mid-July, Dan decided to take a trip to the Black Butte Ranch in Central Oregon, visiting with his two sons at a friend's house. He told me they planned on some "mountain stuff," including fly fishing and climbing. When I called him for our interview, the Winter men had just returned after hiking more than 8 miles along the Metolius, considered by some to be the most magical of all Oregon rivers. I felt myself shiver as Dan commented, "Although nobody's saying it aloud, I suspect it has occurred to my boys that this is probably the last time the three of us will be able to do these things."

Dan had forgotten our appointment, and he didn't recognize my number when I called. I texted him, and we were then able to connect. "Outdoorsy stuff" held little interest for John, who was content to remain at home in Portland with their dog. Dan's daughter was attending summer school, and she also couldn't come.

Dan and I talked about the current deliberations regarding the timing and method of his demise. About the former, he was carefully weighing family circumstances and the progression of the Alzheimer's. He knew that the symptoms in early-onset dementia can suddenly and rapidly crescendo—"avalanche" was the word he used—and that he couldn't afford to wait too much longer. It had been 4 years since the diagnosis, and he was aware that his condition was noticeably worsening.

The previous day, Dan called his mother, who "reiterated that it is *not* an option for her to outlive me.... She was joking a little bit," he said, "but it's obvious she really doesn't want to survive me. I don't blame her."

"Yeah," I said, while feeling a pang of dread about the situation.

"But she's probably not going to have much choice in the matter."

"Yes."

Dan sadly remarked, "I'm not responsible for everybody's reaction. The combination of the disease ramping up and COVID [swirling around] have left me feeling like this is out of my control. Every part, except for the actual act, seems out of my control. I am doing something that's going to have a dramatic impact on people who are the closest to me. I'm making a decision to do something that is going to cause them a lot of hurt. While everybody *gets it*, that doesn't make anyone feel good about it."

Dan had read the soliloquy about suicide by the protagonist in Hemingway's *For Whom the Bells Tolls*: "Anyone has a right to do it, he thought. But it isn't a good thing to do. I understand it, but I do not approve of it.... Sure I understand it but. Yes, but. You have to be awfully occupied with yourself to do a thing like that."[3]

At the Black Butte Ranch, Dan tried to discuss the thorny situation with his sons, and he decided, "They *get it*, but they're not quite hearing it." He guffawed while telling me that he did much of the cooking and how, "One evening during a conversation with my older son, I said, 'You know, it looks like I need to start rounding up some dates.' Tom thought I was talking about making a desert.... Upon realizing the mistake, we all started laughing ... it was a sweet moment." He continued, "But the point of the trip was to address this. I didn't want to talk about it, but I really had to."

Dan was trying his best to sort out his feelings and do what he perceived to be the right thing. He said, "I'm maybe making it a little harder for myself to think that I can keep everybody from feeling bad. Right? I am trying to separate out the 'feeling bad' that you are taking your life and going to be dead, from the fact that you have this terrible disease and if you don't take your life then it's going to continue."

He was able to discuss the quandary with John, and he tried speaking with his therapist, but Dan felt that "even my therapist has caution in his voice when he's talking to me about the subject." Dan said, "It is an almost impossible task.... When it comes to deciding on the day. It's really me alone."

At which point, we had to pause the interview when he accidentally spilled a glass of water on the floor and needed to clean up the mess.

---

[3] Ernest Hemingway, *For Whom the Bell Tolls* (London: Arrow Books, 2004), 350.

Upon resuming, Dan described how he was considering making a videotape for his last day that would be modeled after Sandy Bem's letter. After identifying himself on the recording, he would emphasize that he was alone in the apartment, why he had chosen to kill himself, and that he had not been coerced or influenced by anyone. He would have liked the company of others but realized the situation called for him to step out on the ice floe by himself and drift away.

15

Dan was increasingly more aware that his command of language was slipping. This was certainly evident to me during each of our successive telephone sessions. It was one of the reasons that I arranged to interview John a few days after each conversation I had with Dan. But, in addition, I appreciated hearing John's perspective and found myself growing fonder of both men.

Dan began noticing that people frequently didn't understand him when he spoke; however, most were too polite to ask for clarification. Accordingly, he began speaking less often.

In addition, John observed the onset of a new and odd mannerism—Dan would occasionally reach up and grasp his own head, "as if he was trying to keep parts of his brain from leaking out."

The two men had just returned from a four-night trip to Missoula, Montana, where they met with Dan's three children, his ex-wife, Wynne, and their various partners. The setting was pristinely beautiful—a cabin on Flathead Lake, located right near the entrance to Glacier National Park. The house's deck was suspended over the water, and each night the Winter clan unwound to indescribably beautiful sunsets. The setting was perfect for their intimate gathering.

According to John, "The family made up their own version of Bingo, which they called *Dango*. It was all about Dan. It was a splendid opportunity to tell stories about Dan accompanied by much raucous laughter.

"But," he also observed, "it was sometimes a bit overwhelming for him. Conversations that once would have had his hearty participation left him silent. He was exhausted by the end of each day. He is aware of things changing. It is sobering."

However, this did not stop Dan from cooking breakfast while joyously accompanying a Whitney Houston recording of "I Will Always Love You," with its introductory lyrics, "If I should stay / I would only be in your way / So I'll go, but I know / I'll think of you every step of the way."[1] He loudly sang along with

---

[1] Whitney Houston, "I will always love you," Genius.com, accessed November 20, 2022, https://genius.com/Whitney-houston-i-will-always-love-you-lyrics.

Whitney, vigorously whisked eggs, and awkwardly danced around the kitchen. Later in the day, Dan had vanilla ice cream—his favorite—which he regularly stocked in the fridge. According to John, "Mostly, everybody was very up, and they were funny, brash, and loud. Really just delightful."

Yet, as Whitney's lyrics suggested, death—or at least leave-taking—was a subtext on everyone's mind. They each discussed their willingness to be present when Dan took the lethal cocktail. But after that point the logistical details became blurred. Were people going to assemble in the same room and wear masks? Was it understood that they couldn't safely hug each other? Would they sit on the terrace of the condominium together in the fresh air or would they clump around at the bedside? Would Dan go to his bedroom and each of them then enter separately for a final goodbye? Would it be appropriate to drink champagne?

However, in the morning, Dan said to his husband, "I'm back to wondering if it should just be you and me."

John nodded his head and thought, *I'm so glad he's thinking that way.*

Dan had watched films and read about individuals who choreographed their deaths and organized "living wakes," inviting friends and intimates for a final embrace and creating elaborate, bittersweet rituals with carefully selected music, poetry, food, and liquor. Sandy Bem's circle of loved ones had handled her suicide in exactly that way. But while he correctly considered himself to be quite sociable, this idea didn't appeal to Dan—especially during the pandemic. He wouldn't have minded having a few visitors—except that John was immunocompromised from HIV. In this time of the COVID virus, Dan also didn't want his children or others to undergo the dangers of travel. He especially preferred to avoid anyone facing the possibility of criminal risks related to his death—although he thought this highly unlikely in progressive Oregon.

By the conclusion of the Missoula trip, Dan was confident that a rational suicide made sense to everyone as being the most reasonable method for him to employ. There would not be a party, but he thought they were now prepared to support him.

*****

"Do you think we should continue to be thinking in terms of a date, or should we be thinking in terms of symptoms?" John asked Dan.

"Of course, we should be thinking about symptoms," was the reply. Upon further reflection, John agreed. But they couldn't easily decide just what symptom should act as the trigger, although both men suspected it might be related to getting lost.

Dan explained to me that he had just had a shattering experience after walking out of a grocery store. For a moment—which felt like an eternity—Dan was stymied. *Which way do I turn to get back to the condo?* he wondered. Although John tried to mollify him that such things could happen to any preoccupied person, Dan was extremely distressed.

I suspect that almost everyone falls into one of two camps: those who are traumatized when they get lost (like me) and those who aren't especially bothered and may even welcome the sensation. The writer Ingrid Rojas Contrerask, who suffered brain damage following an accident, fits into the latter group.[2] She is never quite sure of her location in space, and she has come to rejoice in seeking out mazes and labyrinths. In an essay, Contrerask wrote: "Is it strange that I enjoyed this? It felt like a miracle when I reached my destination. . . . [I] think about what it is I love so much about being lost. It's not the puzzle that interests me but how the bright confusion I feel is besieged by a wonder that multiplies."

At this same time, Dan had also begun having more frequent auditory hallucinations. This symptom can emerge even during the prodromal or mild cognitive impairment phases of the neurodegenerative disease continuum.[3,4] In his case, it was as if people were loudly talking in a passing automobile with the windows rolled down. Dan's impression was that the voices came from behind and were moving. Although he found the hallucinations to be "eerie," he was considerably more upset by his momentary disorientation outside of the grocery store.

John noted that his husband was becoming more frustrated, having increasing trouble retrieving words, and finding himself unable to follow the plot lines of television shows. "Dan," he said, "remains very controlled; we're both living with controlled emotions. Which is not to say that we don't express them, because there are certainly times when we do. It's just that we can't be bleeding all day long."

"Listen," I said, "a naive observer might say about someone who has a dementia that they're not in pain and therefore they're not suffering. You're living with a man who has Alzheimer's disease. You have spoken of his daily frustrations, but do they qualify as suffering?"

"Precisely," he replied, "and the most distressing aspect is his very real awareness of being less of who he has been. I just don't think there's anything more personal and more intimate than being aware of losing yourself. It's not the kind

[2] I. R. Contreras, "Paradise Lost," *Sunday New York Times Magazine*, March 26, 2023, 56.

[3] Zahinoor Ismail, Byron Creese, Dag Aarsland, Helen C. Kales, Constantine G. Lyketsos, Robert A. Sweet, and Clive Ballard, "Psychosis in Alzheimer disease: Mechanisms, genetics and therapeutic opportunities," *Nature Reviews Neurology* 18, no. 3 (March 2022): 131–144, doi: 10.1038/s41582-021-00597-3. Epub 2022 Jan 4. PMID: 34983978; PMCID: PMC9074132.

[4] Roberto Monastero, Francesca Mangialasche, Cecilia Camarda, Sara Ercolani, and Rosolino Camarda, "A systematic review of neuropsychiatric symptoms in mild cognitive impairment," *Journal of Alzheimers Disease* 18, no. 1 (2009): 11–30.

of suffering that those of us who haven't experienced it can put into words. He is literally feeling himself disappear."

"Every few seconds," John exclaimed, "Dan is reminded of what he's not."

John was articulating the difference between physical and existential suffering.[5] While I understand that America's existing assisted dying laws, unlike those found in several other countries, are directly linked to capacity, the imminence of death, and physical symptoms, shouldn't these criteria warrant revisions? Dan, John, and I maintain that people ought to have the right to insist on controlling the end of their lives when life as they know it—when the identity that they have proudly forged—is ceasing to exist. Tate and Pearlman have proposed a model of subjective patient suffering linked to losses, including one's sense of self.[6,7] Dan would have directly related to this type of suffering, and he would have bitterly objected to the outsized role of prognosis—with all its limitations—as being one of the core criteria for American assisted dying.[8]

The previous day, both Dan and John participated in another Compassion & Choice (C&C) webinar. Dan told the story about Wint, his own diagnosis, and why he wanted—why he needed—to manage the end of life. "But then he began to ramble a little bit," John said. "I was successful in redirecting him."

"Good," I said.

Afterward, Dan alluded to John's intervention and expressed his gratitude. John told me, "It was just one more instance of him not being who he wants to be."

Dan remarked to me, "I don't know how much longer I can do this."

After he read these words, Dr. David Grube, who retired from a primary care practice in a small Oregon town and served for several years as the National Medical Director of C&C, wrote to me (August 20, 2022, email), "Those of us who have done this kind of actual hands-on end-of-life practice understand that the enemy is not death. The enemy is intolerable terminal suffering. *That* is the context."

Dr. Grube went on to say: "We clinicians only determine the diagnosis/prognosis, but it is the patient who determines the intolerability and the suffering.

[5] Lewis M. Cohen, *A Dignified Ending: Taking Control Over How We Die* (Lanham, MD: Rowman & Littlefield, 2019).

[6] Tyler Tate and Robert Pearlman, "What we mean when we talk about suffering: And why Eric Cassell should not have the last word," *Perspectives in Biology and Medicine* 62, no. 1 (2019): 95–110, doi: 10.1353/pbm.2019.0005.

[7] Robert A. Pearlman, "Understanding the role of suffering in legalized physician-assisted dying," in Sheldon Rubenfeld and Daniel Sulmasy (eds.), *Physician Assisted Suicide and Euthanasia Before, During and After the Third Reich* (Lanham, MD: Rowman & Littlefield, 2020), 193–206.

[8] Nicholas A. Christakis, *Death Foretold: Prophecy and Prognosis in Medical Care* (Chicago: University of Chicago Press, 2001).

Too often we forget that. We are too focused on the kind or type of her/his death . . . even knowing its inevitability."

*****

John was in his studio when we next connected, but with everything that was going on, he was finding it difficult to create art. He explained, "It's almost two years ago since Dan spoke at the original C&C online fundraiser, and at that time he made it very clear he was thinking about the terminus of life. He didn't say how he would die. . . . The administrators from the nonprofit organization are now aware that he has plans to end his own life, but that's not the subject at this point."

"Correct."

"That'll be a future conversation which I'll have with them because I don't want to complicate their mission. Neither can I participate in anything other than telling the truth about what Dan does."

"That's right."

"And part of my charge is to further that conversation."

"Okay."

"Fight for that right."

I said, "It is pretty clear the organization is going to want to hear certain things from you, and they're not going to want to hear other things."

"Correct," he said.

"And frankly," I said, "this book is being written with an awareness that many of the advocates of the right-to-die movement don't want this subject to be raised now. They don't want the word 'suicide' to be mentioned. They don't want to push for death-with-dignity laws to be more inclusive of people who have dementias or who are not terminally ill—as defined by death within the next 6 months. They would rather put their efforts into doing what they've been doing, which is passing Oregon-type laws in other states and not changing the protocol. This is mainly because they've had sufficient trouble just getting that accepted. They've worked hard to shape the public's support of the basic formula—but adding people with slowly progressive brain diseases who are not imminently dying seems like a big stretch. They are modestly fiddling with the Oregon model, but they are hesitating to make any far-reaching changes."

"Exactly," he replied.

Both of us thought of Sarah Palin, about whom was said, "she was less of a running mate than a running gag."[9] And yet, her "death panel" comment almost

    [9] Matt Bai, "How Joe Biden should solve the Kamala Harris conundrum," *Washington Post*, accessed May 8, 2023, https://www.washingtonpost.com/opinions/2023/05/08/kamala-harris-joe-biden-succession-2024-campaign/.

completely hijacked the public's attention from Obamacare.[10] We remembered Senator Chuck Grassley's inflammatory rhetoric also attacking the insurance program when he said, "You have every right to fear. . . . [You] should not have a government run plan to decide when to pull the plug on grandma."[11] Nothing we were discussing involved a death panel or pulling a plug, but we understood how politicians can turn a phrase and hijack the public's feelings.

I found myself marveling at John's equanimity. I commented on his ability to organize, prioritize, and deal with things in a straightforward manner.

"I don't see any point in making something more difficult than it has to be," he explained. "Early on, I learned how to think practically and bring that into my design career, too. If you're planning on storing the frying pans in a particular kitchen cabinet, then how far do you want to walk to get where you'll keep the spatula?"

John pointed out that of greater importance were his experiences "doing a lot of public speaking about living with HIV." He said, "There are many things that people don't want to hear, unless they're aware that it's coming from someone's heart. Talking about HIV and AIDS in the late '80s and early '90s, it's easy to forget how unwelcome a subject that was. And because I did it fairly easily, I got sent into some of the toughest crowds: the city street workers, the blue, blue, blue-collar guys, who had to be forced into a room to hear somebody give a speech about HIV/AIDS."

John continued with real feeling. "But I saw their faces soften. I saw them hear me. Not all of them, certainly. But there were guys who would come up and talk to me afterward, and others who would run into me at a store, sometimes years later, and they'd say, 'You have no idea what your words meant to me.'"

John first learned that he could deliver hard truths and connect with people when he came out to his dad. "I was 28," he told me. "And I loved what it did to our relationship, which went from being a formal relationship to one where he was comfortable putting his arm around me—something that never happened when I was growing up."

As usual, John and I were talking on the phone, so I could not see his face. But I am confident he was smiling warmly when he said, "My father expressed his respect for me, and how I was living my life and the things that I was doing.

[10] Ben Cosman, "'Death Panels' will be Sarah Palin's greatest legacy," *The Atlantic*, accessed September 26, 2022, https://www.theatlantic.com/politics/archive/2014/05/death-panels-will-be-sarah-palins-greatest-legacy/371888/.

[11] Zaid Jilani, "Grassley scaremongers about government pulling 'the plug on Grandma,'" ThinkProgress, accessed September 25, 2022, https://archive.thinkprogress.org/grassley-scaremongers-about-government-pulling-the-plug-on-grandma-24a95a3c0244/.

A lot of men never get to hear that from their fathers, particularly gay men of my generation."

"Yes."

"Since then, I can express what I feel. I can be entirely honest with Dan, and he responds by being honest with me."

Over the last few months, as I listened to this man and to his husband, I was in awe of their spontaneously humane and caring qualities. They truly loved each other. Although John tried to prepare me that he would cry during our interviews, I didn't anticipate how often my own eyes would brim with tears. I was amazed at how well matched the two men were, and how together they were facing the depredations of Alzheimer's and difficult end-of-life issues.

John finished by saying, "In Missoula, hard stuff had been said, and we left with joy in our hearts."

16

Massive wildfires in September temporarily halted the protests in Portland, but not before the city was wracked by more than 100 consecutive nights of disturbances.[1] The wildfire season had begun in July, and, by its conclusion, over 1 million acres were torched, making it one of the most destructive in Oregon's history. The state's social unrest had also not been entirely quelled and continued to flare up.

Demonstrators marched throughout the city each night targeting different police buildings and other symbols of capitalism and so-called colonialism. Daylight would reveal spray-painted slogans and statues that had been pulled down. In August, a man was yanked from his pickup and brutally assaulted. A video recording of the incident went viral. At the end of the month, a pro-Trump car caravan that entered downtown Portland ended with the killing of a supporter of the right-wing Patriot Prayer group. Several days later, the suspected shooter died when Federal task force members attempted to arrest him in Washington, DC.

Responding to the unrest, the city police department stepped back and federal law enforcement assumed a greater presence. Ahead of the presidential election, the governor ordered the Multnomah County Sheriff's Office and Oregon State Police to assume charge of public safety.[2] Over the next year, the Portland Police Bureau would again attempt to manage the political violence, but it would cite staffing shortages as the reason for its frequent inability to separate groups of anti-fascists, like the Proud Boys, and far left demonstrators, like Antifa.

---

[1] Gillian Flaccus, "Portland's grim reality: 100 days of protests, many violent," *AP News*, accessed September 29, 2022, https://apnews.com/article/virus-outbreak-ap-top-news-race-and-ethnicity-id-state-wire-or-state-wire-b57315d97dd2146c4a89b4636faa7b70.

[2] Maxine Bernstein, "Oregon State Police, Multnomah County sheriff to lead police response in Portland during election, with National Guard on standby," *The Oregonian/OregonLive*, accessed September 29, 2022, https://www.oregonlive.com/portland/2020/11/state-police-multnomah-county-sheriffs-office-to-command-police-response-in-portland-during-election-with-national-guard-on-standby.html.

In September, John composed a letter that he sent to Dan's ex-wife, Wynne, and their daughter and sons. It read:

Dear Family,

When Dan and I met with you four, I said that I'd be willing to send you occasional updates on the progression of Dan's illness. I haven't. I think you've all either seen Dan often enough or spoken with him enough to get a sense of the progression. At least I hope so. But things seem to be changing more quickly in the last couple of months and I feel like I need to describe to you what I see happening. Forgive me if I'm over-explaining things you've also observed . . . .

[John then mentioned several of the symptoms.] They seem like small things in isolation, but during the course of a day, those events occur with increasing frequency, so more and more of each day is filled with more and more anxiety and frustration. Cooking and baking have long been Dan's salvation as his disease has progressed, particularly during the pandemic. But now, those activities which have been the sources of joy and fulfillment and stimulation are now also becoming the sources of anxiety and frustration. And dread, I fear.

Dan may well have described to you the sensation he experiences more and more of being less of himself. This isn't something that occurs to him every now and then but is becoming ever-present. He's said he feels dumb, or at least dumber.

There are some physical symptoms that have begun to appear like dropping things, clumsiness. I know that he hasn't started from a place of great gracefulness physically . . . but now there are frequent times when things in the kitchen are dropped or bumped into. Again, these aren't things that bother me, I couldn't care less if they weren't symptoms of disease progression. For Dan they are more experiences which produce added anxiety and frustration.

So, while none of these are terribly significant in isolation, they add up to being constant reminders of the inevitable. The window during which Dan is capable of deciding for himself the why and when he is going to end his life is shrinking.

The day Dan came home after getting the test results that showed he had significant cognitive impairment, he sat me down and told me the test results. A central part of that conversation was his absolute conviction to end his life on his own terms. In the nearly 4 years since then, he has never wavered in that conviction. Not once. When we do have conversations about this, I always remind him that he can change his mind about ending his own life. If he did, I would always be there for him. And he knows all of you would be too. Again, he has never wavered.

As the window of opportunity closes for Dan, it means he gets closer to deciding when to end his life. I struggle like you do to keep my desire to have him in my life for as long as possible from coloring what my job in his journey is—to support his decision. Not too long ago, I asked him some stupid question about how and when he thinks about his decision. He looked at me and said, "I think about it all the time." And of course, he does. I do, too. You do, too. . . . And what he is thinking about all the time is not the whether of it all. Just the when of it.

As the day approaches, I will continue to offer him the chance to change his mind. I do not try to talk him out of his decision. I have not and I will not. I do want him to always have the opportunity to change his mind. There has never been a time when he seemed to move in that direction. There has only been certainty.

From the beginning, Dan has said that he wants to die being able to experience love. I can tell you that his ability to express his love for me and for all of you has not lessened. Quite the opposite. I don't know if you have any idea of how deeply he loves and respects all of you, and of his always growing pride in you . . . .

If this brings up any issues or thoughts or concerns, don't hesitate to contact me. And, just FYI, Dan will have read this before I have sent it to you. I want it all on the table . . . .

With much love,

John

When I read John's letter, I was struck by his gentle insistence to Dan's family that they respect his wish for a dignified ending.

In *Inevitable*, Katie Engelhart's superb collection of conversations sparked by the right-to-die movement, the journalist reflects on how "dignity" pervades modern end-of-life discussions.[3,4] She writes: "I can see a unifying thread. It is that people find dignity in authenticity. They find it in consistency and equilibrium and a kind of narrative coherence. It mattered to the people I met that they lived as themselves, as they defined themselves, until the very final moment, even if it meant sacrificing days or weeks or years of life. It mattered how their

---

[3] Katie Engelhart, *The Inevitable: Dispatches on the Right to Die* (New York: MacMillan, 2021).

[4] Terry Gross, "Inside the fight for the right to die: Logistical and ethical challenges," Fresh Air, NPR, accessed September 29, 2022, https://www.npr.org/sections/health-shots/2021/03/09/975175847/inside-the-fight-for-the-right-to-die-logistical-and-ethical-challenges.

lives wrapped up. In this way, a chosen death became a kind of authorial act. It let a person play herself out, until the end."

Dr. Harvey Chochinov makes a similar point in his textbook, *Dignity Therapy*, where he writes, "Maintaining usual routines and living day to day—as long, and to the extent, possible—are ways of clinging to the familiar and, therefore, not relinquishing what we know and, ultimately, who we are."[5]

But there are implicit quandaries in Engelhart's "authorial act" and Dr. Chochinov's observation about people's wish to not relinquish who they are. Madeline Li, MD, PhD, a clinician scientist in the Department of Supportive Care at Princess Margaret Cancer Centre in Toronto, explained that medical assistance in dying (MAiD) providers like herself are intimately aware that their patients may drastically change from the illnesses and medical treatments.

One such phenomenon, Dr. Li clarified (interview on October 18, 2021), is not widely discussed but occurs especially among persons with neurological diseases who are determined to die and uncertain as to when to die.[6] Dr. Li said: "I see this commonly in patients with brain tumors. I'm dealing with a patient now who is facing this exact dilemma, who keeps moving his date for MAiD forward month by month. He loses physical function from the brain lesion and wants assisted dying, and then his steroids are increased, which temporarily shrinks the tumor. He [feels more like himself and] then holds off formally requesting MAiD, and the cycle repeats. It's agonizing for his wife and family."

And to further complicate matters, Dr. Li appreciates that dignity is not a simple, unitary phenomenon. There is basic human dignity (the intrinsic value of all human beings), social dignity (being recognized and respected by others), and personal dignity (how self-worth is subjectively experienced). While Dan clearly felt all these types of dignity had been marred by his Alzheimer's, I believe it was the last that pained him the most.

In my exchanges with Dr. Li, she raised what I consider to be yet another fundamental but unanswerable question: "How much of yourself do you have to lose before the balance of suffering becomes greater than any pleasure you can still experience?"

Complicating matters, the "new" personality evident during a dementia or terminal illness may not necessarily be entirely unpleasant or dysphoric; people may also sometimes change for the better or experience gratification and joy in the throes of a medical disorder.[7] Sandra Bem's family, for example, were

[5] Harvey Max Chochinov, *Dignity Therapy: Final Words for Final Days* (New York: Oxford University Press, 2012), 25.

[6] Tharshika Thangarasa et al., "A race to the end: Family caregivers' experience of medical assistance in dying (MAiD): A qualitative study," *Journal of General Internal Medicine* 37, no. 4 (March 2022): 809–815.

[7] Wendy Mitchell and Anna Wharton, *Somebody I Used to Know* (New York: Ballantine Books, 2018).

delighted by the unexpected nurturing behavior that she lavished upon her new-born grandchild.

Dr. Li and others struggle over which "authentic self" really matters: the "then-self" or the "now-self."[8,9] On one hand, she told me there is "the person you were as you drafted your advance directives [before receiving the diagnosis of Alzheimer's disease] and couldn't imagine tolerating the indignity of diapering." On the other hand, there is "the person facing the MAiD practitioner now, who seems to be content and is tolerating the diapering just fine."

Belgian oncologist Jan Bernheim, MD, PhD, helped establish the first palliative care unit on the European continent, and he is a professor of medicine and medical ethics at Vrije Universiteit Brussel Faculty of Medicine. He translated for me an opinion piece (interviews on April 24 and May 1, 2020) in which he had written: "First of all, one must make a vital distinction: there are at least two types of deeply demented people: the miserable and the cheerful. The former are cramped, show painful grimaces, struggle against care, and sometimes refuse food. In the best-case scenario, already now [they] are benefiting from a reduction in suffering by not receiving treatments that would prolong their suffering lives. Mind you, this is standard practice, just good paternal care, regardless of whether the demented patient has written a disposition about it. On the other extreme you have the evidently blissful [individual with] dementias who fully enjoys 'a pee, a poo and porridge.' This can be a person who in the past has clearly asked for euthanasia when she or he would get into that condition. Very few doctors would likely give euthanasia to someone like this. Not so much because doctors' values are above the (earlier) wishes of the patient, but precisely because doctors want to serve the current values of their patients. After all, they are no longer the values that he/she adhered to at the time of the advance directive of euthanasia, but they now consist in fully enjoying an extremely shrunken life. It is no longer the same person who made the advance directive, but a very reduced person. And doctors and other caregivers do not have the person of the past, but the person of today as a patient."[10,11]

[8] Andrew D. Firlik, "Margo's logo," *JAMA* 265, no. 2 (1991): 201, doi: 10.1001/jama.1991.03460020055013.

[9] Katie Engelhart, "The mother who changed: A story of dementia," *The New York Times Magazine*, accessed May 10, 2023, https://www.nytimes.com/2023/05/09/magazine/dementia-mother.html.

[10] Jan Bernheim, "Volstaat pisje, poepje, papje om voort te leven?," *De Tijd*, November 26 2019, https://www.tijd.be/opinie/algemeen/volstaat-pisje-poepje-papje-om-voort-te-leven/10185542.html.

[11] Jan L. Bernheim and Kasper Raus, "Euthanasia embedded in palliative care: Responses to essentialistic criticisms of the Belgian model of integral end-of-life care," *Journal of Medical Ethics* 43, no. 8 (August 2017): 489–494, doi: 10.1136/medethics-2016-103511.

Dr. Li would go on to tell me, "I have seen competent people adjust to previously unimaginable circumstances, and the blessing of dementia is the frontal
lobe impairment that induces apathy."

Dr. Benzi Kluger, founding director of the Neuropalliative Care Service
and Palliative Care Research Center at the University of Rochester School of
Medicine and Dentistry, questions whether "apathy" is the appropriate word
for this phenomenon, and he suggested to me (October 9, 2022, interview)
that "anosognosia" is probably a more suitable, technical term.[12] This involves
deficits of insight or self-awareness, and it is defined as being the inability of
neurological patients to recognize their own cognitive, behavioral, or functional impairments. An example of this was when Dan thought he had "aced"
the diagnostic battery of neuropsychological tests.[13,14] Anosognosia can be a
problem—and would have been if Dan continued to believe he was safe driving
behind the wheel of his car—but it also can allow people to have a better than
expected quality of life with dementia. It can help them cope and adjust to unimaginable situations.

First identified back in 1914 by the celebrated neurologist Joseph Babinski,
more recent imaging research into anosognosia and dementia highlight the
specific involvement of medial temporal lobe structures, in particular the right
hippocampus.[15,16] Dr. Kluger adds that, "There are also differences in left versus
right hemisphere involvement which can correlate with emotional regulation.
Personality effects are similarly complex and likely involve multiple nodes in
different brain networks."[17]Anosognosia's severity increases with disease progression. Subjective complaints of depression tend to decrease, while inhibition

[12] Eric Ecklund-Johnson and Ivan Torres, "Unawareness of deficits in Alzheimer's disease and
other dementias: Operational definitions and empirical findings," Neuropsychology Review 15, no. 3
(September 2005): 147–166, doi: 10.1007/s11065-005-9026-7.

[13] Filomena Galeone, Stella Pappalardo, Sergio Chieffi, Alessandro Iavarone, and Sergio
Carlomagno, "Anosognosia for memory deficit in amnestic mild cognitive impairment and
Alzheimer's disease," International Journal of Geriatric Psychiatry 26, no. 7 (July 2011): 695–701,
doi: 10.1002/gps.2583, Epub 2010 Dec 23, PMID: 21495076.

[14] S. Sevush and N. Leve, "Denial of memory deficit in Alzheimer's disease," American Journal of
Psychiatry 150, no. 5 (May 1993): 748–751, doi: 10.1176/ajp.150.5.748, PMID: 8480820.

[15] J. Babinski, "Contribution a l'étude des troubles mentaux dans hémiplégie organique cèrébrale
(anosognosie), trans. Karen G. Langer and David N. Levine, Cortex 61 (December 2014): 845–847,
doi: 10.1016/j.cortex.2014.04.019.

[16] Manuela Tondelli, Anna M. Barbarulo, Giulia Vinceti, Chiara Vincenzi, Annalisa Chiari, Paolo
F. Nichelli, and Giovanna Zamboni, "Neural correlates of anosognosia in Alzheimer's disease and
mild cognitive impairment: A multi-method assessment," Frontiers of Behavioral Neuroscience 12
(2018): 100, doi: 10.3389/fnbeh.2018.00100.

[17] Benzi Kluger, accessed October 14, 2022, https://benzikluger.com/.

of socially unsuitable behaviors become more problematic as anosognosia worsens.[18]

Apathy? Anosognosia? I would add a third word that likely has a bearing on how people and their caregivers cope with dementing illnesses, and that is "denial." Denial is a defense mechanism in which an individual refuses to recognize or acknowledge objective facts or experiences.[19] It's an unconscious process that serves to protect the person from discomfort or anxiety. The concept arose mainly from the work of the pioneering child analyst Anna Freud and her father, Sigmund Freud.[20,21]

According to Professor Emerita Joan Berzoff from the Smith College School for Social Work (March 4, 2023, interview): "Defense mechanisms, like denial, are unconscious strategies that people automatically employ to shield themselves from anxiety and other distressing emotions by rejecting aspects of reality. All defense mechanisms have the potential to be protective or pathological. Denial is manifested when individuals are confronted by situations or truths that threaten to be overwhelming, such as the acknowledgment of addiction and substance abuse."

However, Professor Berzoff says, "Often the basic human will to survive is more powerful than any self-destructive impulse, mightier than any defense, and stronger than any disease."

Given that Alzheimer's is among the most feared health condition in America and the United Kingdom,[22,23,24] it is hardly surprising that denial is pervasive among those diagnosed with dementias. The above neuropsychological,

[18] Yukiko Kashiwa, Yurinosuke Kitabayashi, Jin Narumoto, Kaeko Nakamura, Hideki Ueda, and Kenji Fukui, "Anosognosia in Alzheimer's disease: Association with patient characteristics, psychiatric symptoms and cognitive deficits," *Psychiatry and Clinical Neuroscience* 59, no. 6 (December 2005): 697–704, doi: 10.1111/j.1440-1819.2005.01439.x, PMID: 16401246.

[19] "Denial," Psychology Today, accessed February 13, 2023, https://www.psychologytoday.com/us/basics/denial.

[20] A. Freud, *The Ego and the Mechanisms of Defense* (London and New York: Routledge, 2018).

[21] Sigmund Freud, "The loss of reality in neurosis and psychosis," in James Strachey (ed.), *The Standard Edition of the Complete Works of Sigmund Freud, Vol. 19* (London: Hogarth Press, 1961), 183–187.

[22] "What medical condition are you most afraid of?," Medicare Advantage website, accessed April 17, 2023, https://www.medicareadvantage.com/news/most-feared-heath-conditions-report#:~:text=The%20Top%205%20Most%20Feared,%2C%20strokes%20and%20COVID%2D19.&text=Cancer%20fears%20are%20more%20than%20justified.

[23] Dan G. Blazer, Kristine Yaffe, and Jason Karlawish, "Cognitive aging: A report from the Institute of Medicine," *JAMA* 313, no. 21 (June 2015): 2121–2122, doi: 10.1001/jama.2015.4380.

[24] "Over half of people fear dementia diagnosis, 62 per cent think it means 'life is over,'" Alzheimer's Society, accessed October 8, 2022, https://www.alzheimers.org.uk/news/2018-05-29/over-half-people-fear-dementia-diagnosis-62-cent-think-it-means-life-over.

neurological, and psychopathological mechanisms likely coexist and are implicated in the person's lack of awareness of deficits.[25] I believe they contribute to people accommodating and accepting their neurodegenerative disorders.

Dan is one of the exceptions. It is worthwhile examining why he continues to be so determined to take action when most people with dementia develop a tolerance for the burdens and limitations imposed upon them by their slowly progressive illness. I suspect that the process by which he came to acknowledge his childhood sexual abuse and addiction, and the manner in which he came to accept his homosexuality, plus his experience observing the enormity of his father's losses all helped him to recognize and perhaps be less controlled by denial and the related phenomena.[26]

And yet it warrants stating that even Dan hadn't effectively prepared to end his life before he sat down in the neuropsychologist's office or until after he had met with the neurology consultant. There are things that he might have done years before (e.g., information he might have acquired, membership established in right-to-die organizations like Final Exit Network, as well as specific items and equipment he could have acquired to better arrange for his death). But it is basic human nature to accept and not effectively take steps in preparation for the forest fires that erupt each summer in Oregon.

[25] Raphaël Trouillet, Marie-Christine Gély-Nargeot, and Christian Derouesné, "La méconnaissance des troubles dans la maladie d'Alzheimer: Nécessité d'une approche multidimensionnelle [Unawareness of deficits in Alzheimer's disease: A multidimensional approach]," Psychol Neuropsychiatr Vieil 1, no. 2 (June 2003): 99–110, PMID: 15683946.

[26] K. G. Langer, "Depression and denial in psychotherapy of persons with disabilities," American Journal of Psychotherapy 48, no. 2 (Spring 1994): 181–194, doi: 10.1176/appi.psychotherapy.

17

In October, Dan paid a quick visit to his elderly mother in Kansas City, but the trip unfortunately triggered the tall man's always delicate orthopedic situation, which had originally required three separate surgeries. Exacerbated by an uncomfortable airline seat, Dan was writhing with back spasms when John met him with a wheelchair at the Portland airport gate. Dan would spend nearly 3 weeks at home in forced hibernation, unable to walk or bike around the neighborhood. He was only able to finally obtain relief after receiving a steroid injection.

During this time, his short-term memory was noticeably worse, and he felt crushing fatigue. He was more aware of the hallucinations and emotional irritability.

When I spoke with Dan, he had a "silly question" for me: "This is ridiculous," he said, "but I'm going to ask it anyway. Do you think there's a hospice that would take me for my last couple of days? A residential hospice?" He then went on to say, "However, nobody's going to do that for somebody who's killing himself. Right?"

"Mmm-hm," I muttered.

Dan then mused, "So, has life gotten to be *not* worth living?" And he immediately answered his own question, "No, not yet."

Like John, Dan had written a missive—a group email—that would eventually be sent to friends, thanking them for having made a difference in his life. He had also come up with a list of a dozen people whom he intended to phone as the terminus approached.

Dan's thoughts were scattered, and he recapped his visit to Flathead Lake with the declaration: "The kids are just taking it and treating it very well. I have no idea how their reaction will be after I die. But I think that I've done all I can in getting them to understand." He then wistfully remarked, "They've supported me from the beginning."

For now, he was mainly staying at home and trying to minimize further back spasms. He stalwartly resisted taking any pain medications because of his history of drug abuse.

"I don't have access to Oregon's Death with Dignity Act," Dan said, "for very good reasons: practical, ethical, and political. But I'm still curious why there's not going to be any accommodation for a patient like me with Alzheimer's for a number of years."

"I've been speaking with some people in the Netherlands," I said, "and the Dutch law would include someone like yourself."

"Yeah, I thought about going there," Dan said.

"You did?"

"I did. It was one of my options, but I got comfortable with the fact that I could administer this myself with support from John."

Listening to his response, I refrained from pointing out that he would not have been eligible because he wasn't Dutch, and he was probably thinking of Switzerland. That liberal country *would* have accepted him under its law, which permits "suicide tourism" (a grotesque phrase) for people with either terminal illnesses or those suffering from chronic, unendurable conditions, such as dementias. This is well described in Nan Weiner's *Los Angeles Times* piece about her mother-in-law's assisted suicide at the Dignitas clinic, in which she recalls: "We even laughed about the fact that once we all arrived in Zurich, hers was the only luggage that didn't make it. (Believe it or not, it finally showed up the day she died.)"[1]

Globally, the Netherlands and Belgium have instituted detailed processes to permit people with dementia to access voluntary assisted dying since the early 2000s, and the federal government of Canada created a legal protocol in 2016, which it is continuing to refine as evidenced by the assisted death of Wayne Briese.[2] Meanwhile, Luxembourg and Colombia are developing procedures to permit access by people with these conditions, and currently in the Netherlands and Belgium, even the loss of mental capacity from late-stage dementia does not make a person entirely ineligible for assisted dying once he has completed the application process.[3] Medical assistance in dying (MAiD) practitioners in these

---

[1] Nan Weiner, "Opinion: The story of my mother-in-law's assisted suicide," *Los Angeles Times*, accessed May 8, 2023, https://www.latimes.com/opinion/story/2023-05-07/assisted-suicide-right-to-die-law-dignitas-alzheimers-dementia.

[2] Sheila Wayman, "Assisted dying: 'I do not want to end my days as a lost soul in a nursing home': One couple's story of four years from dementia diagnosis to assisted death," *The Irish Times*, accessed September 26, 2023, https://www.irishtimes.com/health/your-family/2023/09/26/assisted-dying-wayne-if-life-is-a-stage-how-do-you-want-to-take-your-final-bow/.

[3] Roy Harvey, "Australia's voluntary assisted dying laws don't really allow dying with dignity," *Canberra Times*, accessed May 14, 2023, https://www.canberratimes.com.au/story/8193846/its-not-really-dying-with-dignity-in-australia/.

countries rely on a "Ulysses contract," based on the Greek hero's instructions to his sailors to fill their ears with wax and tie him to the mast so that they would not be affected while he might hear the sirens' fabled singing.[4,5]

Likewise, in June of 2023, the legislature in Quebec voted overwhelmingly in favor of an *advance request* measure to expand its program of assisted medical death.[6] People affected by a cognitive neurodegenerative disease who are in the earlier stages, like Dan, could request an assisted death for up to 24 months later—when they then no longer had capacity. According to Georges L'Esperance, president of the Quebec Association for the Right to Die with Dignity, "With advance requests, people affected by a cognitive neurodegenerative disease who want medical assistance in dying can finally have a peaceful end of life." A petition before the Canadian House of Commons has more than 16,000 signatures, and according to the Council of Canadian Academies Colombia, Spain and the Netherlands all allow advance requests, while Belgium and Luxembourg allow these when the person is unconscious at the time of the procedure.[7]

Voluntary Assisted Dying laws were recently enacted in all of the Australian states, and the public is requesting that these be extended to include people who have dementias. In October 2023 draft legislation endorsed by the human rights commissioner, children's commissioner and disabilities commissioner was introduced to the Australian Capital Territory's parliament.[8]

When I connected again with John, he was in his art studio, preoccupied with an elaborate black-and-white drawing that resembled to my eyes a sandworm's mouth in the Frank Herbert novel, *Dune*. John confirmed that Dan and he had briefly contemplated going to Switzerland for aid in dying, but the two men eventually rejected this option because, "It felt like we were running away."

*****

[4] Andrea Daverio, Gioia Piazzi, and Anna Saya, "[Ulysses contract in psychiatry]," *Riv Psichiatry* 52, no. 6 (November-December 2017): 220–225, doi: 10.1708/2846.28725.

[5] Adam D. Marks and Judith C. Ahronheim, "Advance directive as Ulysses Contract: The application of stopping of eating and drinking by advance directive," *American Journal of Hospice and Palliative Care* 37, no. 11 (November 2020): 974–979, doi: 10.1177/1049909120912951.

[6] David Ljunggren, "Quebec allows sick patients to request assisted death in advance," *Reuters*, accessed June 9, 2023, https://www.reuters.com/business/healthcare-pharmaceuticals/quebec-allows-sick-patients-request-assisted-death-advance-2023-06-08/.

[7] Rebecca Zandbergen, "Should dementia patients be able to make advance requests for medical assistance in dying?" CBC News. Accessed February 13, 2024. https://www.cbc.ca/news/canada/ottawa/dementia-patient-maid-canada-request-rules-1.7101508

[8] World Federation of Right to Die Societies. Australia: HRC seeks expansion of VAD. January 12, 2024. https://wfrtds.org/australia-hrc-seeks-expansion-of-vad/

Dan was more animated than usual when we spoke next.

The couple were the featured storytellers at another annual event sponsored by Compassion & Choice (C&C), which was attended this time by 800 people. During the Zoom webcast, they again refrained from either explicitly talking about the decision to foreshorten life by a pharmaceutical overdose or their thoughts about voluntary dying laws. Once again, their emphasis was focused on the organization's initiative to encourage completion of enhanced advance directives—"dementia directives"—to prevent lives from being artificially extended. These documents focus on withholding and withdrawing life-prolonging treatments and delineating how the individual wishes caregivers to manage nutrition when the disease progresses to the point that one ceases evincing any further interest in eating. At the meeting, Dan told the audience, "I'm glad to be able to talk about the dementias and end-of-life planning in the same sentence."

When he and I spoke later, Dan was pleased with what he called, "a hidden agenda" within the American right-to-die movement, "to provide people, like me, a seat at the table to take advantage of the medical aid in dying protocol . . . while we still have some cognitive capacity to dictate on paper what we will and won't live with."

However, Dan then contradicted himself and said that he wasn't happy "when states put together death-with-dignity legislative programs or ballot measures. It's always been understood that these would be hands-off for people with dementia or Parkinson's . . . a third rail."

Dan reiterated what he had told me 6 months earlier: "I am angry that I have to break a law in order to take my own life. . . . I'm frustrated there is an Oregon aid-in-dying program, and I can't access it. It pisses me off that I have to worry how many milligrams of this or that medication I'll need to take, and in what particular order. I'm resentful. But at the same time, I completely understand."

"Tell me more," I said.

He replied indignantly, "It's still going to be years before there will be any legal or political attempt to include people like me in medical assistance in dying. Maybe along the way someone will say, 'Oh yeah, I remember Dan Winter talking about how the Holy Grail of the movement is to figure out a way to allow people like him—folk with Alzheimer's disease—to access the system instead of going on their own.'"

Dan then brought up the subject of Brittany Maynard, the 29-year-old Californian who had a glioblastoma of the brain and was prominently featured in *People* magazine.[9] She had posted several videos online that went viral. He said,

[9] Nicole Weisensee Egan, "Terminally ill woman Brittany Maynard has ended her own life," *People*, accessed March 17, 2023, https://people.com/celebrity/terminally-ill-woman-brittany-maynard-has-ended-her-own-life/.

"Brittany had the opportunity to use her fantastic pulpit to emphasize death with dignity for people who are suffering with cancer, and I think she did a huge service to the movement. I would love to think that my situation, even if in just a small way, could advance the conversation . . . maybe get people to find ways for those who want to end their lives when they have one of the dementias? I hope there are people who look at my example and say, 'That guy was a semiregular person.'"

"A semiregular person? Okay. . . . "

"I don't have any special features," Dan continued. "I'm not particularly brave. I'm not particularly well-spoken. I'm not particularly smart. God, I would just be so. . . . " His voice trailed off.

When he resumed, Dan said, "If anybody uses my situation as a part of the reason that they could die the way they want to—that would be a huge compliment."

I suggested, "That you could be an inspiration, the way Brittany Maynard was for so many people, and you could help to change the laws?"

"Yeah, absolutely. I'd love it if I was remembered for taking my own life because of dementia," he concluded.

Thus prompting my colleague, Peter A. DePergola II, PhD, MTS, Chief Ethics Officer at Baystate Medical Center, to write (May 2, 2023, email) about the irony of Dan wanting to be recalled while "managing an illness that prevents him from remembering."

*****

"We've had some *interesting* issues around his family," John exclaimed. Earlier, the conversation appeared to have gone well when Dan had traveled to Missoula to talk to the children and their mother. They seemed supportive of Dan's terminal care preferences and understood that he didn't want anything done to prolong his life, such as artificial feeding or other medical interventions. He was explicit with them that his intention was to overdose if he stayed physically healthy but continued to mentally fail.

Then John sent his letter to the core family members, underscoring Dan's plan. Word spread throughout the extended clan that he was going to take his life before the end of the year. Neither of the two men fully or accurately anticipated the family reaction. According to Dan, "The letter broke the dam." As it dawned on the Winters that the year was coming to a close, a few members began heatedly expressing their uncertainty about the wisdom of such an action. Dan received calls in which individuals made statements like, "Gee, you're doing great. You don't need to think about this yet!"

John told me that the interactions were "unsettling, and they weren't constructive." Dan felt disrespected and was unpersuaded. He thought the primary reason the family had problems with the plan was because some of them hadn't directly witnessed his mental and physical deterioration and were therefore not ready to let him go.

John summarized: "We're getting calls, and they don't want it to happen now. They love him. I don't really blame them. But it takes energy for us to respond. I had prepared Dan for this because it's akin to what I experienced when people found out that I was HIV positive. It's true of anybody who gets a serious diagnosis—the patient ends up consoling friends and family members. So, Dan isn't entirely surprised, although it's difficult to navigate."

One of Dan's acquaintances pointedly remarked, "You don't owe these people anything in terms of how they're dealing with this. Please don't feel like you're going to be excoriated after your death if you didn't get around to calling everybody."

This exact same opinion had also been expressed by Susan Dunn,[10] a 59-year-old Canadian woman who, with a few weeks remaining before her scheduled death by MAiD, said she wanted to make every second count and didn't want to waste time thinking about her decision not to inform all her family and friends about the details.

"I'm having enough trouble from now to then keeping my shit together," Dunn wrote. "I hope my friends understand, but for me to call up every person I love and say, 'Hey this is what I'm doing,' and say, 'Goodbye!' it's too hard and I would just fall apart."

John agreed with Dunn's conclusion. "But this is Dan's thing," he said. "How he deals with it is exactly how he chooses to deal with it. This is the most personal, intimate, and consequential decision-making process that a human can undergo."

John and Dan then asked me to "keep off the record" identifying information about individual family members whose reactions were distressing them. It was the only such request that they made during our many hours of interviews. John said, "I don't want you to write about who in the family has been resistant to the plan."

Writers are constantly called upon to make ethical choices, and I have never forgotten Janet Malcolm's finger-wagging words, "Every journalist who is not too stupid or too full of himself to notice what is going on knows that what he does is morally indefensible."[11] Especially during this writing project, there

[10] Jennifer Hamilton-McCharles, "North Bay mother of two ends life on her terms," *The Sudbury Star*, accessed July 23, 2022, https://www.thesudburystar.com/news/provincial/north-bay-mother-of-two-ends-life-on-her-terms-2.

[11] Janet Malcolm, "The journalist and the murderer: What is journalism for?," *The New Yorker*, accessed May 29, 2023, https://www.newyorker.com/magazine/1989/03/13/the-journalist-and-the-murderer-i.

were distinct moments in which I thought about my responsibilities as an author and contrasted them with my erstwhile roles as a psychiatric professor, medical provider, and palliative care researcher. Those other jobs were considerably simpler.

For example, I was aware that the use of amitriptyline in DIY overdoses—like Dan was planning—is occasionally associated with a highly uncomfortable burning sensation in the mouth and throat. It can last for several minutes until the person becomes unconscious. But the discomfort can be easily ameliorated if one has been instructed in advance about chewing on a popsicle or swallowing some nonfat sorbet. Knowing that Dan intended to use this medication placed me in a quandary: Should I bring up the complication? Ought I to inquire whether Dan and John had heard about the simple management technique and were prepared? While I decided to not explore the topic, I remained troubled.

Likewise, I had recently learned that the addition of phenobarbital (a barbiturate anticonvulsant) reportedly decreases the time to death and improves the reliability of other aid-in-dying medications. Was this a topic I should raise, or would I then be actively facilitating rather than merely reporting on Dan's suicide? Again, I chose not to broach it or discuss the specifics of the medication cocktail. I figured that if I was an embedded combat reporter, I ought not carry a weapon and begin shooting. But I was uncomfortable with my decisions.

However, when John and Dan invoked their "off the record" request regarding the family, I had considerably less difficulty. Admittedly, compelling tales are always enhanced by the presence of rogues: the Sackler's, Jeffrey Epstein, Elizabeth Holmes, and Professor James Moriarty in Sherlock Holmes come to mind. Naming specific family members would have heightened the dramatic qualities of Dan's story. But, upon reflection, I did not feel by acceding to the couple's request that my integrity as a journalist would be compromised.

I spent a fair amount of time discussing the matter with both men and was reassured by John, who remarked, "The good news is that in this case there are no real villains—only a few people whose hearts aren't ready yet. That's been hard for us."

In a conversation, Dan made it explicit that he didn't want individual family members who disagreed with him to be identified because he loved all of them. He suspected that such disputes are almost inevitable in situations like his own. He very much *wanted* the issue of family conflicts to be articulated so others could read about this, anticipate it in their own futures, and make decisions accordingly.

In this context, Dan and I revisited the role of the Winter clan in the "Bleeding Kansas" period before the Civil War—that time of turmoil and violence when it was uncertain whether the territory was going to enter the Union as a slave state or a free state. According to Dan, while his family wanted to think of themselves as having uniformly been abolitionists, as a young man who was interested in journalism, he had interviewed his two favorite great-aunts. "They were sisters," he explained, "and they were arguing about whether their own father and uncle were secret slavers or open free staters." Dan pointed out to me that the present conflict over him committing suicide was hardly the first time that the Winter family was likely divided by intense moral issues.

I commented, "It must be fascinating to belong to a family that appreciates the longevity and complexity of its personal history."

He responded, "It sure beats talking about one's outrage over country club scandals."

And I guessed that this had also been the subject of occasional Winter household conversations.

18

While I assumed that the issue of whether family members should be invited to Portland for a final visit had been settled, this was apparently not the case. Instead, the two men continued debating between themselves. But the issue was finally resolved when I spoke next with John, who declared, "So, it will be Dan and me and Friday."

"On a Friday?" I asked.

"No," John replied. "Friday's the dog." At that moment, I heard some barking in the background.

"Oh! My mistake!" I realized that his name had come up before, but I didn't recall anything about him. "What kind of dog is he?" I asked.

"*She's* a 28-pound Labradoodle."

"How old? How did she come into your life?"

John replied, "She is just 7 years old, and we got Friday in 2013, when we moved into our house."

"And how has she now adjusted to apartment living?"

"Very well," John said. "She's a great dog. Labradoodles have a reputation for being smart, well-behaved animals, and she just fits the bill. Friday pays attention, and it makes life easy. We refer to her as 'the love factory.' Dogs are a wonderful life force, and she has been very important to Dan. At this period when Dan is much more reflective because of the back pain he's been having, she doesn't leave his side. I take her to the park where she does what she needs to do, and when we come back, she just can't wait to get in the door and run to him."

"So, in the end, it will be the three of you?" I asked.

"Yup."

"And when Dan is dead, what's next?"

John explained, "He is donating his body to Oregon Health & Science University—the research medical facility here in town. I'll be giving them a call."

"Because someone has to declare him dead and all that sort of thing . . . ," I mumbled.

"Somebody from the university comes and deals with the legal part before they take the body," said John. But a thought crossed my mind, *I hope they are not being overoptimistic about the process.* However, I was impressed that Dan had chosen this selfless act—to become one of the estimated 20,000 whole-body donors whose contributions help American students in anatomy laboratories.[1]

"John," I said. "In my most recent interview with Dan, I asked him, 'Are you sure you want to be talking to me? For that matter, *why* do you want to talk to me?' And Dan had replied, 'Because I want people to hear about this. I want to open up the subject so other people can converse about it.'

"John, does that jibe with what you are hearing from him as well?"

"Oh, certainly," he said. "We share that motivation. I have wondered recently about what happens to me after Dan dies. I can't know the answer other than that grief will have its way. But I need something else to give added meaning to my life and have wondered, *Is this it? Is this subject a thing that I will want to continue to deal with and to promote?*"

Until that conversation, I hadn't specifically thought about John's anticipatory grief. I was preoccupied with the immediate issues, but John knew quite well that, without Dan, his identity was going to drastically change. After 10 years of being married, his future, his very self, would metamorphosize into something entirely new.

*****

Dan began our next interview with a couple of flip comments about the implications of the national 2020 election results on his Republican family members. But then he quickly shifted and announced his decision to kill himself during the second week of January. His symptoms were continuing to progress, and he somberly declared, "This disease is an exercise in things being removed from you."

The tall man sighed: "My communication with people, other than John, even my siblings and my kids, are less satisfying to me," he said. "I feel myself not wanting to be in the discussion because I'm not able to get *it*—whatever *it* is that we're talking about. I know those people who are closest to me can tell, and I hear them try to modulate what they're saying and make it easier for me. They slow it down.

---

[1] April Rubin, "Honoring the body donors who are a medical student's 'first patient,'" *The New York Times*, accessed June 4, 2023, https://www.nytimes.com/2023/05/31/science/donor-bodies-medical-school-appreciation.html.

"I was a journalism major, then I became a bank president, and then the director at the ACLU. In all those roles, I was expected to be prepared and to make remarks that were germane, and helpful, and sensitive, and thoughtful, and maybe even funny and colorful, all of them depending upon the situation. Now, I can't communicate."

I should interject at this point that, throughout this book, I've liberally been using my editorial license in smoothing over linguistic and grammatical problems with Dan's quotes. Some of them were evident in our first interview, but they worsened each month. At one point in writing this manuscript, he and I paused and then reviewed the quotes to make sure they still accurately reflected his thoughts. I also later checked them with John and confirmed that I was accurately recording his own statements.

At this point, Dan was finding that phone calls from friends and family had become exhausting. According to John, "Dan would work so hard to be 'Dan' during a call, that afterward he would drop and hold his head in his hands."

Basic communication had become laborious, and Dan told me, "The inability to communicate is one of the things that I don't want to live with. I don't want to live in a world where I can't understand what people are saying."

Nursing authority Diana Waugh offers the following analogy: "Have you ever driven down the road into a fog? In a nanosecond what happens? You think to yourself, *If I slow down will somebody hit me from behind? If I go too fast, will I hit somebody? Am I in the right lane? Did I pass my exit?* Fifty million thoughts go running through your mind. I don't know if this is true or not, but . . . having memory loss is like constantly living in that kind of a fog."[2]

I continued to listen to Dan ruminate, and he explained that a malaise which used to set in for him at 5 PM each day was now starting at 2 PM. If he was chopping an onion in the kitchen when this occurred, he was liable to accidentally injure himself. John and he agreed that his symptoms were becoming intolerable, and the second week of January was sufficiently far enough away from Christmas that Dan's death wouldn't be associated by his family with the holiday.

During our last couple of interviews, the man's disorganization and concentration impairment were considerably more prominent. Dan would occasionally comment on these and apologize whenever he lost track. Our conversations jumped from him talking about his 87-year-old mother's Catholicism and her resistance to accepting his end-of-life plan, to what it was like as an adolescent listening to the OK Ranch cowpokes gossiping about the whore houses on Ninth

---

[2] Diana Waugh, "How to talk to someone with dementia," mmlearn.org, accessed November 15, 2022, https://www.youtube.com/watch?v=ilickabmjww.

Street outside of Fort Riley, to the moment he and his wife told the children that he was gay and they were getting divorced.

Dan's scattered thinking was also evident when he tried to address the subject of his addictive behaviors, which had begun in high school and then steadily worsened. When Dan was an adult attending social and professional events, upon returning home he would continue unabated drinking. This went on, he said, until his wife, Wynne, finally confronted him. One night, she declared, "You've talked to your counselor about it, but you aren't changing. If you're not going to commit yourself to quit drinking by your birthday or you say you're going to do it and then don't. . . . Well, you're out of here!"

"And that," Dan explained, "is not only how I attained sobriety, but also one of the many reasons why I greatly love and admire my wife."

The "clear-headedness" that followed sobriety contributed to him summoning the courage to cease lying to his therapist and to finally begin talking about having been raped. "And that changed everything, because I had not divulged this to anyone and had depended upon an entire structure of denial around it for myself."

Dan said that he came to terms with the abuse by allowing his story to be posted online, and "I told everybody I could about the circumstances. I drove or flew to each of my four siblings, got in front of them, and told the story. I was very systematic and process oriented about it."

In that same year, he also realized "I couldn't hide I was gay anymore." The epiphany was followed by the couple deciding to continue their marriage for a while longer. Dan and Wynne accepted that there would come a time to separate and divorce, and they knew and regretted that their children would suffer the consequences.

One of Dan's most transformative experiences occurred with his psychologist, who inquired, "When are you going to begin forgiving yourself and face the shame and guilt of the childhood sexual abuse?"

Dan was struck dumb.

After a suitable pause, the therapist then asked, "Now tell me again, how old were you when this happened?"

"Twelve."

[Incidentally, when Dan originally told me about the attack, he said that he was fifteen.]

The psychologist probed, "How old are your children now?"

"Fifteen, twelve, and nine."

He followed up by inquiring, "Would you blame your twelve-year-old son if he was abused?" The therapist waited, but Dan was stunned again into silence by the question.

The psychologist then asked, "If not, why are you continuing to blame yourself?"

And this exchange apparently broke a significant emotional log jam.

*****

"Do you have sufficient medical care at this point?" I asked Dan.

"I tell any physician that I see about the Alzheimer's, but there isn't any active treatment. There are only two medications that may slow it down, and one of them wasn't helpful for my dad. There's really nothing to treat. The only thing that physicians agree will slow—but not halt—Alzheimer's is regular exercise. So, I've been on an intense exercise regimen and have cleaned up my diet."

At this point, my colleague, Canadian psychiatrist Harvey Chochinov, might very well have questioned whether Dan had lost hope, any sense of meaning, or purpose.[3] Dr. Chochinov would have inquired whether Dan felt that he no longer mattered. And my colleague might have questioned whether a therapeutic intervention was warranted.

But, in my opinion, Dan was a realist. He instinctively understood the difference between hope, acceptance, and denial. In our interview, he summed things up by saying, "I'm a relatively happy human and I'm enjoying my life now. There's a huge, dark cloud in it, but I'm going to finish this telephone call and go see the guy who married me."

I inquired, "And that makes you feel?"

"Grateful. I have all these incredible people around me, and I'm sorry that I'm not going to be able to spend more time with them. But I'm so grateful having people who I love and who love me. I have had a wonderful life."

Later, John also spoke to me about hope: "I wouldn't say I'm spending much time hoping, because hope doesn't change the course of anything. In this circumstance, I think hope can be blinding or can at least obscure the reality that's standing right in front of you. In some circumstances, there's a place for hope. I am not hopeless about very many things. It's probably semantics, but for me there's a difference between not having hope and being hopeless."

John concluded, "Hope is about the future, and delight is in the moment. We choose not to invest in hope around Dan's Alzheimer's and that is serving us well."

*****

[3] Harvey Max Chochinov, "Intensive caring: Reminding patients they matter," *Journal of Clinical Oncology* 41, no. 16 (June 2023): 2884–2887, doi: 10.1200/JCO.23.00042, Epub April 19, 2023.

I asked Dan if there were any people whom I might interview to get a more three-dimensional picture of him and his life. Interestingly, one of Dan's recommendations turned out to be his psychoanalyst, a psychologist named Dr. David Donovan from Kansas City, who originally began working with him some 15 years earlier and who reconnected after the Alzheimer's diagnosis.

The takeaway from our subsequent interview (November 30, 2021) was that Dr. Donovan noted Dan's cognitive slippage and that he was having a harder time finding words; however, the clinician felt his patient remained very thoughtful and rational about the plan to kill himself. He had never previously made a suicide attempt, and his substance abuse remained completely under control. "Something I find very touching," the psychologist said, "is that he's revisiting the past a lot more in this wistful, nostalgic way, but he doesn't seem depressed at all. He's kind of enjoying remembering the good times, and he's playing them over in his head."

Dr. Donovan found it heartbreaking when Dan told him about his inability to keep up with conversations and how he'd been pulling away from people. Although Dan had gone through a period of depression decades earlier, "by his nature, he is a very upbeat and dynamic person." If the Alzheimer's had affected his mood at all during the past 4 years, it had contributed to making him "seem more content and kind of calmer." Dr. Donovan was confident that Dan was not presently depressed.

Pausing to collect his thoughts, he told me, "Dan's an extraordinary man who's had an extraordinary life. I think that he's touched many people, and it's been amazing what he's done."

19

Dan settled on January 15 as the specific day that he would overdose.

"I had an experience, last week," he explained to me, "which made me realize the time is right. I was at the park where I take the dog at least twice a day."

It's a very conventional, old-fashioned kind of park—big-tree lined sidewalks and grassy areas and wooden benches—a beautiful, tranquil, leafy oasis located just three blocks away from the apartment. It has plenty of places where dogs can relieve themselves. It is the sort of park where thoughtful owners responsibly carry small plastic bags to clean up afterward.

Upon arriving, Dan had bent down to tie his laces. "When I lifted up my head," he said, "time, immeasurable, stopped. I might as well have been in Toledo, Ohio."

This was far worse than the episode that had taken place outside the grocery store of transient mental fogginess. Now, everything around him went silent; all he could hear was the sound of his own breath, inhaling and exhaling, and the rapid beating of his heart. He felt entirely dissociated from ordinary reality. He couldn't recall how he had gotten there or how he would be returning home. Nothing looked familiar.

Dan explained, "It was disorienting to the point that I thought I was going to pass out. . . . I sat down on a bench and let Friday off of the leash."

Both the dog and his master then remained motionless, frozen in place. It may have been 1 minute, or 5 minutes, or 10—he had no way of knowing.

If you have ever dislocated an arm, the pain is immense until the moment it is popped back in place. And that was Dan's experience. With no forewarning, he popped back. Suddenly, time resumed, and the park was instantly identifiable. Standing up and grasping the labradoodle's leash, he stumbled—partly in shock and partly because his balance has lately been more impaired—back to the condominium.

In Wendy Mitchell's memoir about her vascular dementia and young-onset Alzheimer's disease, there is a frighteningly similar episode in which she, too, is outside, standing on a familiar street corner, when suddenly the mental fog descends upon her and she recognizes nothing.[1] Mitchell writes: "I get a coffee and stare out at the square I know so well but which had been lost in an instant. How did that happen? A short circuit in my brain, a disconnect somewhere between my eyes. I'm reminded that this disease can steal the past, the present and the future."

And then, like Dan, the fog abruptly lifts for Mitchell, and she shuffles back through her accustomed streets to home.

How would a neurologist understand what happened? When I asked Dr. George Naasan (October 27, 2022, interview), he said that Dan may have had a small seizure, or perhaps he experienced a "fluctuation" of Lewy body disease, or perhaps the not uncommon Alzheimer's phenomenon of disorientation and inability to navigate one's environment.[2]

Concerning the latter, Dr. Naasan explained: "Most of the time this happens for reasons that have to do with the way the brain is processing visual cues and the environment. You and I take it for granted that if you're in a restaurant and you go to the restroom, your brain is memorizing how you got there. You know, 'I got up from my chair and I walked straight to the back, and then I made a left, and then there were stairs going down, and when I reached the bottom of the stairs, I made a right. Yes, and then the bathroom was there.' We take all of that for granted. Somehow after we've finished washing and drying our hands, we come back and magically find the table without even batting an eyelash. You know, we don't even think about it. But for a person with Alzheimer's disease, it can be an unmanageable task. They are lost because the moment they leave the bathroom, they are uncertain as to whether they turned right or left. They are unclear about the location of the stairs. They are unsure whether that was the hallway. Getting lost with Alzheimer's has more to do with the brain's inability to memorize visual cues, to hold on to information that you just received through your eyes, to no longer automatically lay down a mental map."

John was at home when Dan arrived. He walked in the door with Friday, and his expression was one of pure alarm. John would later tell me, "The blood had drained from his face and there was terror in his eyes. He was deathly pale, and I knew something unusual had happened. I got out of my chair immediately and quickly walked toward him."

Dan's hands were trembling as he exclaimed, "I have fallen into the void."

[1] Wendy Mitchell, *Somebody I Used to Know* (New York: Ballantine Books, 2018), 140–141.

[2] J. Bradshaw, M. Saling, M, Hopwood, et al, "Fluctuating cognition in dementia with Lewy bodies and Alzheimer's disease is qualitatively distinct," *Journal of Neurology, Neurosurgery & Psychiatry* 75, no. 3 (March 2004): 382–387, doi: 10.1136/jnnp.2002.002576.

When I heard about Dan and the park, it made me realize that we probably underestimate the extent of discomfort experienced by people who have dementing illnesses. There is a popular misconception that they become pleasantly confused. Unlike cancer, patients don't routinely complain of pain, itching, or nausea. Neither are they grossly disfigured by a tumor or by surgery. And, at a certain point, they cease talking entirely. We are then left only to imagine what they are experiencing. While *we* suffer when the personalities of loved one's dissolve, perhaps we need to appreciate more the magnitude of *their* suffering and that it may be infinitely greater than our own. In many instances, it is likely a rationalization on our part that they have adapted to their circumstance.

But who knows? Perhaps for most people with neurodegenerative disorders the elemental pleasures become more enjoyable as the brain atrophies and their world shrinks? Perhaps the increased caring and outpouring of affection from family members outweigh any potential discomfort about being a burden? Perhaps. . . .

For individuals with dementing illnesses, the marker for intolerable suffering is very individualistic. Kevyn Morris, 62, an advisory committee member for Dementia Australia who was diagnosed almost 7 years ago, wrote, "If I get to the point where I'm a head in a bed or I'm sitting at the window in a princess chair, drool running down my cheeks, not knowing if I'm Arthur or Martha—that's not, that's not a life for me. That's, that's cruelty."[3]

"If you were a horse, you would be put down and no one would blink an eyelid," Morris told a reporter.[4]

Back in 2019, Gayle Garlock became one of the first Canadians with dementia to receive medical assistance in dying (MAiD).[5] According to his wife, the retired university librarian and scholar, who was diagnosed with Lewy body dementia, the second most common form of memory disorder after Alzheimer's disease, found continued life to be unendurable after he lost the ability to read.

I know of another individual who sought death when she was on the cusp of requiring placement in a nursing home, concerning which geriatric psychiatrist

[3] Bianca Iovino, "'With dementia, you've already lost them': Voluntary assisted dying laws reviewed," HelloCare, accessed May 26, 2023, https://hellocare.com.au/with-dementia-youve-already-lost-them-voluntary-assisted-dying-laws-reviewed/.

[4] M. Cunningham and H. Cook, "It kills almost 10 per cent of Australians: But dementia patients have no say in how they die," May 21, 2023, accessed May 28, 2023 https://www.smh.com.au/national/it-kills-almost-10-per-cent-of-australians-but-dementia-patients-have-no-say-in-how-they-die-20230518-p5d9gm.html.

[5] "B.C. man is one of the first Canadians with dementia to die with medical assistance: A person with dementia who meets the MAID criteria should be eligible, doctor says," CBC Radio, October 27, 2019, https://www.cbc.ca/radio/sunday/the-sunday-edition-for-october-27-2019-1.5335017/b-c-man-is-one-of-the-first-canadians-with-dementia-to-die-with-medical-assistance-1.5335025.

Brent Forester commented (August 23, 2023, interview), "Families are often re-luctant to make the decision to move someone into a long-term facility, and it's often because that person had said at some point in time, 'Well, I never would want to live there.' Yet, once the decision is made and mom or dad or spouse goes to the assisted living or the long-term care facility, I never hear families saying, 'Oh my God, what a mistake.' Instead, 99.9% of them say, 'Why did I wait so long?'"

I also knew of an elderly naval officer who decided to die after becoming in-continent of stool. And on the subject of incontinence—which is very common in dementia—is it really so bad?

Professor Catherine Frazee and I spoke (December 11, 2022), and she has written: "Having to wear diapers and drooling are highly stigmatized departures from what is expected of adult bodies. Those of us who deviate from these norms"—and she was talking about herself and many others in the disability community—"experience social shame and stigma that erodes resilience and increases vulnerability. The more deeply these stigmatized accounts are embedded in our discourse and social policy, the more deeply virulent social prejudice takes hold within our culture."[6]

And if Professor Frazee's observation is upsetting to hear, well, let's also at-tend to the words of her colleague, Gabrielle Peters, who said: "It is not a hard stretch for any of us to understand how you can then conclude that the world would be better without you and that the lives of people around you would be better without you. That is exactly . . . the rational conclusion . . . based on the things we're being told by the society we live in."[7]

Add to this the observations by Drs. Foley and Hendin that "Physicians con-sistently underestimate the quality of life of patient who have disabilities,"[8] and Alexiou's position that a death-hastening practice—and he was specifically fo-cusing on MAiD—"devalues the divergent but meaningful lived experience of disabled people and provides the state with an easy way of foregoing its responsibilities to its most vulnerable citizens."[9]

---

[6] Catherine Frazee, "'The vulnerable': Who are they?," Canadian Virtual Hospice, accessed December 18, 2022, https://www.virtualhospice.ca/en_US/Main+Site+Navigation/Home/For+Professionals/For+Professionals/The+Exchange/Current/%E2%80%9CThe+Vulnerable%E2%80%9D_+Who+Are+They_.aspx.

[7] James Wilt, "Filibustering death-dealing ableism: An interview with Catherine Frazee and Gabrielle Peters on the Disability Filibuster and Bill C-7," Canadian Dimension, accessed December 2, 2022, https://canadiandimension.com/articles/view/filibustering-death-dealing-ableism. June 2, 2022.

[8] Kathleen Foley and Herbert Hendin, The Case Against Assisted Suicide: For the Right to End-o-Life Care (Baltimore: Johns Hopkins University Press, 2004), 316.

[9] Gus Alexiou, "Canada's permissive euthanasia laws spark debate on the true meaning of disa-bility," Forbes, accessed January 10, 2023, https://www.forbes.com/sites/gusalexiou/2023/01/10/

Dr. Paul Lippmann (d. March 14, 2022) has suggested that incontinence is not necessarily bad if there are others willing and available to clean one up afterward.[10] When the elderly, erudite, 86-year-old psychoanalyst (who did *not* have a dementia) fractured his femur, requiring months in a hospital and rehabilitation center following surgery, he observed, "I was being cared for in the most intimate fashion in my body, in my mind, in my soul. The nurses, their assistants, physical and occupational therapists, cleaning personnel, food preparers and deliverers, the doctors, all were cleaning, washing, and wiping me, and changing the bed linen when I soiled myself, and feeding me, and trying to make sure, day and night, that I was not in any distress or discomfort. To my surprise, during all this intimate handling of my infirm naked body, I felt absolutely no sense of embarrassment or shame, something that ordinarily would have forced me to cover up, hide, and make sure no one witnessed my naked, disordered, infantile loss of control over bodily functions."

Dan never reached that point in the final stage of Alzheimer's where such support is necessary because for him the excruciating experience of becoming disconnected in space and time was his marker of intolerability. It powerfully reinforced his long-held wish to comply with Nietzsche's maxim: "Many die too late, and some die too early. Yet strange soundeth the precept: 'Die at the right time!' "[11]

Getting lost at the neighborhood park was Dan's marker, his trigger, his personal nightmare come to life. Why was it so traumatic? The answer possibly resides in the "cognitive map: hypothesis from neuropsychology and neuroimaging, which Edward C. Tolman first suggested 75 years ago.[12] This hypothesis proposes that the brain constructs a unified representation of the spatial environment to support memory and guide future actions.[13] From early childhood onward, people make sense of themselves in relation to the physical world by processing information spatially. Other animals make use of a similar mapping processes, as witnessed by the scent-marking of territory performed by dogs or the dance of the honey bee.[14] Recognizing landmarks and navigation are central

canadas-permissive-euthanasia-laws-spark-debate-on-the-true-meaning-of-disability/?sh=dd8e7 992aa0c.

[10] Paul Lippmann, "On getting old," *Contemporary Psychoanalysis* 58, no. 1 (2022): 103–111, doi: 10.1080/00107530.2022.2095187.

[11] Friedrich Nietzsche, *Thus Spoke Zarathustra*, "Voluntary Death," 4umi.com, accessed December 18, 2022, http://4umi.com/nietzsche/zarathustra/21.

[12] Edward C. Tolman, "Cognitive maps in rats and men," *Psychological Review* 55, no. 4 (1948): 189.

[13] R. A. Epstein, E. Z. Patai, J. B. Julian, and H. J. Spiers, "The cognitive map in humans: Spatial navigation and beyond," *Nature Neuroscience* 20, no. 11 (October 26, 2017): 1504–1513, doi: 10.1038/ nn.4656. PMID: 29073650; PMCID: PMC6028313.

[14] Jerry Brotton, *A History of the World in 12 Maps* (New York: Viking, 2012), 8–9.

to our identities, and when people become untethered from the world, it can be devastating. For Dan, this signaled that the right time to die had arrived.

*****

Dan began reaching out to core members of his family, notifying them of the date he had selected. He declared in a straightforward way that he could no longer bear life with dementia any longer. On one hand, he welcomed death and the freedom it offered. On the other hand, he was devastated at the thought of leaving his beloveds behind. He wanted each of them to understand the decision was only reached after painful consideration. But, at the same time, it had clicked into place and made perfect sense to him and to John. He was insistent they must let him go.

By the end of December, word had spread among the 17 members of the Winter clan who Dan used to regularly text, and they were urgently speaking with each other. Most were accepting of Dan's choice and his right to take his life. But some balked, and they asked: Is it true you're not being followed by a neurologist? How come you aren't seeing the nation's expert on Alzheimer's or taking part in a clinical research study? Why aren't you taking a dementia medicine? How about another MRI? Why kill yourself in the middle of January? Wouldn't it be a simpler matter to wait until Z graduates? Can't you postpone until X or Y occurs?

John was contacted by a skeptical relative who inquired, "Why don't you just wait until Dan can no longer feel joy and love, and then tell him, 'It's time to die?'" Another emailed John and requested, "How about getting him to wait just a few more days?"

John uncharacteristically snapped, and he wrote back to both, "This isn't like changing an airline reservation!"

Professor Frazee, who has spinal muscular atrophy, a hereditary disease that progressively destroys motor neurons, appreciated the family's queries. She explained to me: "I hold that we don't actually own our lives. We share our lives and life. If we think of this as a resource or a gift, it is only a gift insofar as it is shared and has meaning for others as well as ourselves. . . . Plus, dementia can open up pathways to new forms of flourishing that are not rooted in privilege or power."

"Not so," wrote Michael T. Bailin, MD (April 20, 2023, email), Chairman Emeritus from the Department of Anesthesia at Baystate Medical Center: "I do believe we have agency over and control our lives. Seeing patients over the years with unremitting terminal illness pain, or hearing people with end-stage dementia screaming in the hospital while on night call, I can't imagine myself in that bed. I want a better ending than that. Maybe when one is no longer able to care for themselves, Professor Frazee's 'shared lives and life' is front and center. But presuming that every person wants (in advance) or should go on living with crippling dementia in a bedbound, paralyzed state, dependent to toilet, eat and dress, is another story."

Dan had predicted and dreaded these conflicting reactions. "I've explained to everybody this is a game in which you must give up good time, and there's no way to know how much good time you're giving up. So, the game is not to try to find the perfect date, because that's a game you'll lose."

It was this mantra that he repeated to his dear ones.

But, like Ruth Oppenheim's family, who didn't want to hear that she intended to overdose rather than succumb to dementia, and who would later write: "Then for a while we all tried to do this impossible thing, which is to try to tether someone to life when they are moving away, tying knots in the ropes of love and memory while they are just as busily untying them."[15,16]

Oppenheim's daughter sorrowfully explained: "I had assumed that at the end of the day my mother would do the conventional thing. That she would go on living, until forced out of life by a failing body. But she was not conventional in that way. She was unpredictable. She acted by her own rules, not those of others. She decided on her own way. I had misjudged her so terribly."

Dan fully understood that his relatives were speaking about the disease from a place of love—and also one of ignorance and denial—but why, he still wanted to know, would they not accept his judgment and appreciate that he had considered all of these matters? Was it because he had a dementia and they thought he was not to be trusted?

John tried to reach out to settle the "family kerfuffle" by offering additional information. He gave them further examples of how Dan was deteriorating and suffering. But he was frustrated because to the family skeptics, Dan's imminent suicide—rational or not, and whether or not that is the correct word to use—represented an embarrassing tear in the social fabric. For some of them, it was contrary to fundamental moral and religious beliefs.

John Swinton, a professor of practical theology and pastoral care at the University of Aberdeen, has written: "[Dementia] isn't something that is internal to an individual's neurological makeup ... the self remains intact even in the most severe forms of dementia." Elaborating on this theme, he continued, "Any loss of self relates to a failure of community. Everything we have and everyone we know

---

[15] Natasha Walter, "My mother planned her own death for a long time: Why didn't I believe her?" *The Guardian*, accessed August 20, 2023, https://www.theguardian.com/books/2023/aug/20/mother-planned-own-death-natasha-walter-before-the-light-fades-suicide.

[16] Natasha Walter, *Before the Light Fades: A Memoir of Grief and Resistance* (London: Virago Press, 2023).

exists because of God and is deeply loved by God . . . human beings are both wanted and loved irrespective of their physical or psychological condition."[17,18]

In the same vein, the Evangelical Fellowship of Canada, like many other religious organizations and some faith-based healthcare delivery systems, adamantly opposes euthanasia and assisted dying.[19] It maintains that "the appropriate response to suffering is to address and alleviate the suffering, not to eliminate the one who suffers. We respond to those who are suffering with care and compassion, journeying with them as they walk in the shadow of death. . . . It is not for us to choose the timing of our death."

While Dan was not seeking a medically assisted death—because his Alzheimer's made him ineligible under Oregon's statute—the spokesperson of the Evangelical Fellowship would have certainly felt the same way about Dan arranging to take an overdose.

"Morally depraved!" is Vancouver Archbishop J. Michael Miller's opinion of Canada's MAiD laws. Montreal Rabbi Berel Bell has likewise declared, "From our viewpoint, every life has equal value . . . but when a life should end is not something that should be left up to human beings. Our Creator knows how and when to end lives, and He does it every day."[20]

Meanwhile, the normally staid *British Medical Journal* published an Islamic commentary with capital letters for emphasis that read: "ASSISTED SUICIDE, SUICIDE AND EUTHANASIA ARE ALL FORBIDDEN IN ISLAM. No one should have the intention to kill himself or herself, even with the assistance of somebody else. There are many verses in the final Holy Book, AL QUR'AN, which emphasize these basic Pro-life Islamic beliefs. If I can quote one verse: 'In the Name of GOD, the Most Compassionate the Most Merciful, DO NOT KILL YOURSELVES, FOR VERILY ALLAH/GOD HAS BEEN TO YOU MOST MERCIFUL' (chapter 4, verse 29)."[21]

---

[17] John Swinton, *Dementia: Living in the Memories of God* (Grand Rapids, MI: William B. Eerdmans, 2012).

[18] Woodruff J. English, "Review of *Dementia: Living in the Memories of God*, by John Swinton," Catholic Health Association of the United States, accessed October 1, 2022, https://www.chausa. org/publications/health-progress/archives/issues/november-december-2014/book-review-dementia-living-in-the-memories-of-god.

[19] "EFC factum version 17 as filed," Evangelical Fellowship of Canada, accessed October 1, 2022, https://www.scc-csc.ca/WebDocuments-DocumentsWeb/35591/FM100_Intervener_Evangelical-Fellowship-of-Canada.pdf.

[20] John Hayward, "Canadian religious leaders speak out against 'morally depraved' euthanasia policy," Breitbart, accessed November 26, 2022, https://www.breitbart.com/national-security/2022/11/23/canadian-religious-leaders-speak-out-against-morally-depraved-euthanasia-policy/.

[21] Majid Katme, "Muslim medical reasons against assisted suicide: Rapid response to: Assisted dying—time for a full and fair debate," *British Medical Journal* 351 (2015): h4517, doi: https://doi.org/10.1136/bmj.h4517.

In 2019, representatives from the Abrahamic religions: Christianity, Judaism, and Islam, signed a joint declaration at the Vatican entitled, "The Rejection of Euthanasia and Physician-Assisted Suicide." They wrote that these practices "fundamentally contradict the inalienable value of human life, and therefore are inherently and consequentially morally and religiously wrong, and should be forbidden without exceptions."[22]

Daniel Sulmasy, MD, PhD, Director of the Kennedy Institute of Ethics at Georgetown University approaches this issue from a somewhat different vantage in his response to an article written by Rutger's Law Professor Norman Cantor.[23] Professor Cantor had explained why, in the event of Alzheimer's, he would want to hasten his own death whether by voluntarily stopping eating and drinking or withholding and withdrawing life-prolonging treatments. To this Dr. Sulmasy replies: "We should never ratify the idea that the world is better off without you even if you come to believe it. We should mourn your loss, not precipitate it. The reason we shouldn't endorse your killing yourself is the same reason you gave in your essay about why we should not let you soil yourself—out of respect for your basic human dignity. You are valuable not only for your intellect but as a fellow human being. Should you develop a dementing illness, we should keep you warm, comfortable, and clean, treat your pain, and care for you."[24]

Interestingly, by way of contrast, the ancient Greeks and Romans, including Sophocles, Zeno, and Pliny, all approved of suicide,[25] with Seneca the Younger famously writing: "Against all injuries of life I have the refuge of death. If I can choose between a death of torture and one that is simple and easy, why should I not select the latter? As I choose the ship in which I sail and the house which I shall inhabit, so I will choose the death by which I leave life. The wise man will live as long as he ought, but not as long as he can."[26,27]

[22] "Position paper of the Abrahamic monotheistic religions on matters concerning the end of life (Casina Pio IV, 28 October 2019)," accessed January 25, 2023, https://press.vatican.va/content/sal astampa/en/bollettino/pubblico/2019/10/28/191028f.html.

[23] Norman L. Cantor, "On avoiding deep dementia," *Hastings Center Report* 48, no. 4 (July/ August 2018): 15–24.

[24] Daniel P. Sulmasy, "An open letter to Norman Cantor regarding dementia and physician-assisted suicide," *Hasting Center Report* (July/August 2018), accessed December 15, 2022, http:// bioethics.pitt.edu/sites/default/files/publication-images/CEPResources/October2018/Sulmasy-2018-Hastings_Center_Report.pdf.

[25] Charles McKhann, *A Time to Die: The Place of Physician Assistance* (New Haven, CT: Yale University Press, 1999), 58.

[26] Seneca the Younger, "Letters," LXX, from "Quotes of Seneca the Younger," Imperium Romanum, accessed May 17, 2023, https://imperiumromanum.pl/en/roman-art-and-culture/gol den-thoughts-of-romans/quotes-of-seneca-the-younger/.

[27] M. D. Sullivan and S. J. Youngner, "Depression, competence, and the right to refuse life-saving medical treatment," *American Journal of Psychiatry* 151, no. 7 (July 1994): 971–978, doi: 10.1176/ ajp.151.971.

The Hippocratic Oath's prohibition against physicians using poison is often cited to further support opposition to euthanasia and physician-assisted dying.[28,29] However, Hippocrates's declaration harkens to a time when doctors were often being asked by aristocratic patrons to use their pharmacological expertise to poison—to assassinate—political rivals and other enemies.[30] In addition, the classic oath shows its age through its opening evocation to Apollo, Aesculapius, Hygeia, and Panacea, as well the proscribing of all surgical procedures and prohibiting of doctors from charging fees for their medical services. There aren't a lot of modern physicians and bioethicists clamoring for these positions.

Not surprisingly, the Hippocratic Oath has been revised numerous times; the version now commonly employed in most US medical school graduations was written in 1964 by Dr. Louis Lasagna. Rather than a list of prohibitions, it includes the following solemn statement: "Most especially must I tread with care in matters of life and death. If it is given me to save a life, all thanks. But it may also be within my power to take a life; this awesome responsibility must be faced with great humbleness and awareness of my own frailty."[31]

During assisted dying debates in the House of Lords, Desmond Tutu, archbishop Emeritus of Cape Town and a Nobel Prize laureate, published an impassioned plea: "In refusing dying people the right to die with dignity, we fail to demonstrate the compassion that lies at the heart of Christian values. I pray that politicians, lawmakers, and religious leaders have the courage to support the choices terminally ill citizens make in departing Mother Earth."[32]

The Churchill Park United Church of Winnipeg, a member of the largest Protestant Christian denomination in Canada, took Archbishop Tutu's words

[28] Leon R. Kass, "'I will give no deadly drug': Why doctors must not kill," in Kathleen Foley and Herbert Hendin (eds.), *The Case Against Assisted Suicide: For the Right to End-of-Life Care* (Baltimore: Johns Hopkins University Press, 2002), 17–40.

[29] Rachita Narsaria, "The Hippocratic Oath: The original and revised version," The Practo Blog, accessed October 31, 2022, https://doctors.practo.com/the-hippocratic-oath-the-original-and-revised-version/.

[30] Franz Lidz, "Scalpel, forceps, bone drill: Modern medicine in ancient Rome: A 2,000-year-old collection of medical tools, recently unearthed in Hungary, offer insight into the practices of undaunted, much-maligned Roman doctors," *The New York Times*, accessed June 14, 2023, https://www.nytimes.com/2023/06/13/science/archaeology-ancient-rome-medicine.html?campaign_id=34&emc=edit_sc_20230613&instance_id=94912&nl=science-times&regi_id=63340269&segment_id=135421&te=1&user_id=895343099129dcd1f95fa65a5a136796.

[31] Narsaria, "The Hippocratic Oath."

[32] Desmond Tutu, "When my time comes, I want the option of an assisted death," *The Washington Post*, accessed October 1, 2022, https://www.washingtonpost.com/opinions/global-opinions/archbishop-desmond-tutu-when-my-time-comes-i-want-the-option-of-an-assisted-death/2016/10/06/97c804f2-8a81-11e6-b24f-a7f89eb68887_story.html.

to heart.[33] In 2022, it became the site of a MAiD ceremony held for one of its members diagnosed with Lou Gehrig's disease (amyotrophic lateral sclerosis). The equivalent of a living wake was convened in the church's sanctuary, and it was there that Betty Sanguin was administered the fatal medication.

The minister reflected afterward, "We were deeply honored to be able to be with Betty in her final moments and hours and to honor her wishes around her dying process. She was so happy, she was so ready, she was so radiant."

It bears stating that neither Dan nor John was especially religious; rather, each of their positions on determining the endpoint of life was secularly based. John understood that some of the Winter family believed the intentional overdose of a man who had a dementia might be acceptable in parts of Oregon but was going to be firmly rejected by most Kansans. But, like the dedicated revolutionaries and abolitionists who preceded them, both men held that individuals should do the right thing and let the consequences take care of themselves.[34] John said with considerable force, "Society hasn't condoned any number of things that only changed because people worked to change them," and he espoused William Lloyd Garrison's position: "I am in earnest, I will not equivocate, I will not excuse, I will not retreat a single inch, and I will be heard. "[35]

However, despite John's persistence, it was apparent to him that the effort to mollify members of the family who objected to Dan's plan was gaining little traction. Some of these individuals couldn't grasp that measures to foreshorten life involving a person suffering from a dementia were not the same as the suicide of a distraught man or woman with a psychiatric condition.[36] Their position obdurately remained, "suicide is suicide is suicide, plain and simple."

Others, like Wynne Winter (December 3, 2022, interview), thought that "knowing Dan, if COVID hadn't happened, I'm certain that it would have been different." She went on to cite the isolation from the pandemic, the difficulties people had adjusting to their changed lives, and that the Winters and their friends couldn't come to Portland and directly engage in a dialogue with her ex-husband. "It wouldn't have been a different outcome," she clarified. "It just

[33] Michael Gryboski, "Canadian church hosts controversial assisted suicide ceremony for member with ALS," *The Christian Post*, accessed October 1, 2022, https://www.christianpost.com/news/canadian-church-hosts-assisted-suicide-for-member-with-als.html.

[34] Lydia Moland, *Lydia Maria Child: A Radical American Life* (Chicago: University of Chicago Press, 2022), 103–104.

[35] "William Lloyd Garrison quotes," Good Reads, accessed May 2, 2023, https://www.goodreads.com/author/quotes/102464.William_Lloyd_Garrison.

[36] C. Creighton, J. Cerel, and M. P. Battin, "Statement of the American Association of Suicidology: 'Suicide' is not the same as 'physician aid in dying.'" American Association of Suicidology, accessed January 21, 2023, https://suicidology.org/wp-content/uploads/2019/07/AAS-PAD-Statement-Approved-10.30.17-ed-10-30-17.pdf.

would've been a different timeline, [and] it would've helped everybody im-
mensely. But not being able to see him. . . . Yes, the big X factor was COVID."

Last, perhaps because they had already witnessed Dan's father accept the care
accorded to a loved one failing from Alzheimer's, some of the family expected
the same acquiescence on the part of Wint's son. And they were disappointed.

Dan was exceedingly unhappy about the pushback and ensuing arguments.
He was plainly irritated, and he bluntly told his family this wasn't a negotiable
matter. Dan wanted them to arrive at a consensus that he had made the correct
decision for himself after carefully weighing the different factors. And he didn't
receive that assurance.

20

Until I heard the objections of the more skeptical members of the Winter family, I hadn't realized that Dan was *not* being followed by a neurologist. I, too, began to wonder: *Was Dan remiss in not having sought out the world's neurological experts in Alzheimer's? Alternatively, should he have volunteered for some cutting-edge Alzheimer's research investigation?* I was puzzled about whether these were legitimate concerns and deliberated, *Just how does the field of neurology presently deal with dementing illnesses?* I pondered about having possibly dismissed the validity of the opposition within the family because of my identification with Dan and John's position.

However, according to Dr. Zachari Macchi, when Dan tried to explain to the skeptics that he had sound reasons for *not* regularly seeing a neurologist, this was probably a valid stance. Many of Dr. Macchi's neurological associates do *not* appreciate that even though the dementias are progressive degenerative conditions, "there's still a lot we can do to manage them." With a broad grin, he told me (October 25, 2022, interview) that the traditional refrain within the specialty has been: "Diagnose and Adios!" Patients may leave the neurology consultant's office having identified and learned a bit about their Alzheimer's or other dementia, but the parting message is often a version of "come back and see me only if things change radically."

Most people's treatment is instead managed by their primary care physician, while a very few are regularly seen by neurologists like Dr. Macchi at outpatient offices or "memory clinics." The latter are new facilities, like Alzheimer's disease research centers, which offer comprehensive multidisciplinary services. They are relatively uncommon and almost always associated with academic institutions.

When I reached out to the director of the memory clinic at Baystate Medical Center, Stephen J. Bonasera, MD, PhD, he turned out to be a gregarious geriatrician and not a neurologist. My assumption had been that the program was primarily intended to establish and fine-tune diagnoses, but Dr. Bonasera describes his model as offering long-term outpatient delivery of services coordinated with primary care providers. The latter group of medical professionals, he explained (December 1, 2022, interview), generally provide most of the follow-up to people with dementias, but "do not have the time to sit down and talk to patients and caregivers about what they are experiencing. They don't have the time to perform detailed medication reviews, identify potentially inappropriate meds, and conduct advanced care planning with their elderly population. They don't have the time to think about the functional status of their patients. They've got 25 minutes in clinic, and that's barely enough time for them to check the blood pressure, do a brief physical examination, and then deal with hypertension medications, type II diabetes, and the most recent new problem to surface."

After arriving at a diagnosis of Alzheimer's disease or vascular dementia or another cognitive disorder, he tells his patients at the memory clinic, "We're now entering into a longer relationship. We're going to get to know each other a lot better in the coming years, but I'll need to check in with you. We need to get comfortable with each other, and to communicate what's going on and what's on our minds. Why? Because our goals are going to change as the situation changes. To really be on top of what you want, we need to be aware of these changing goals and be flexible and able to move when that opportunity arises."

His model is consistent with how geriatricians ideally approach this clinical situation, but also with a new and innovative development that has sprung up among neurologists called *neuropalliative care*.[1]

It has been a quarter-century since the Ethics and Humanities Subcommittee of the American Academy of Neurology issued a statement regarding the need for "neurologists to understand, and learn to apply, the principles of palliative medicine."[2] In 2006, the subspecialty of hospice and palliative medicine was officially recognized by the American Board of Psychiatry and Neurology.[3] It offered an opportunity for a growing number of interested neurologists in the United States and elsewhere—many of whom are among the newest and youngest generation of physicians—to also become board-certified in palliative medicine.[4] These neuropalliative specialists are beginning to practice in hospices, inpatient consult services, memory clinics, and other outpatient programs, and they

[1] Leandro Provinciali, Giulia Carlini, Daniela Tarquini, et al., "Need for palliative care for neurological diseases," *Neurological Science* 37, no. 10 (October 2016): 1581–1587, doi: 10.1007/s10072-016-2614-x.

[2] ""Palliative care in neurology: The American Academy of Neurology Ethics and Humanities Subcommittee," *Neurology* 46, no. 3 (March 1996): 870–2, PMID: 8618714.

[3] Maisha Robinson and Kevin M. Barrett, "Emerging subspecialties in neurology: Neuropalliative care," *Neurology* 82, no. 21 (May 2014): e180–e182, doi: 10.1212/WNL.0000000000000453.

[4] D. J. Oliver, G. D. Borasio, A. Caraceni, et al., "A consensus review on the development of palliative care for patients with chronic and progressive neurological disease," *European Journal of Neurology* 23, no. 1 (January 2016): 30–38, doi: 10.1111/ene.12889.

are focusing on the broad needs of patients and families affected by neurologic disorders, including the dementias.[5,6,7]

Dr. Benzi Kluger explained to me (October 10, 2022, interview) that the palliative care requirements of those who are affected by neurologic illnesses should include discussing goals of care, supporting caregivers, offering spiritual well-being, attending to symptom management, addressing painful emotions such as guilt and grief, and coordinating management with hospices. Around the time that Dan was diagnosed with Alzheimer's, the overall specialty's treatment paradigm began to shift, and neurologists started to become more aware of "significant gaps in the care of patients with neurologic illness in these domains."[8]

The first Neuropalliative Care Summit took place at the 2017 American Academy of Neurology meeting. The Summit proposed that, in addition to the ongoing search to discover cures, it was also necessary to develop better and more comprehensive outpatient care.

Interestingly, Alzheimer's disease and the other progressive dementias offered a particularly difficult challenge to these clinicians.[9] Those illnesses were historically not considered as being appropriate diagnoses for hospice and palliative medical services since they were not thought of as being terminal diseases for many years.[10] Their situation has been exacerbated by the absence of meaningful pharmacological treatments, the pleomorphic pictures of the different types of dementias, the difficulty predicting a trajectory with any exactitude, and the enormous burden the illnesses present to patients and caregivers.[11]

[5] Benzi M. Kluger, Michael J. Persenaire, Samantha K. Holden, et al., "Implementation issues relevant to outpatient neurology palliative care," *Annals of Palliative Medicine* 7, no. 3 (July 2018): 339–348, doi: 10.21037/apm.2017.10.06. Epub 2017.

[6] Lieve Van den Block, "The need for integrating palliative care in ageing and dementia policies," *European Journal of Public Health* 24, no. 5 (October 2014): 705–706, doi: 10.1093/eurpub/cku084.

[7] Jenny T. Van der Steen, Lukas Radbruch, Cees M. P. M. Hertogh, et al, "White paper defining optimal palliative care in older people with dementia: A Delphi study and recommendations from the European Association for Palliative Care," *Palliative Medicine* 28, no. 3 (March 2014): 197–209, doi: 10.1177/0269216313493685.

[8] Isabel Boersma, Janis Miyasaki, Jean Kutner, and Benzi Kluger, "Palliative care and neurology: Time for a paradigm shift," *Neurology* 83, no. 6 (August 2014): 561–7, doi: 10.1212/WNL.0000000000000674.

[9] Charles B. Simone, "The growing challenge of dementia and its impact on patients, their caregivers, and providers," *Annals of Palliative Medicine* 6, no. 4 (October 2017):299–301, doi: 10.21037/apm.2017.07.03.

[10] Ladislav Volicer, "The development of palliative care for dementia," *Annals of Palliative Medicine* 6, no. 4 (2017): 302–305, doi: 10.21037/apm.207.06.12.

[11] Mari Lloyd-Williams, Karen Harrison Dening, and Jacquline Crowther, "Dying with dementia: How can we improve the care and support of patients and their families," *Annals of Palliative Medicine* 6, no. 4 (October 2017): 306–309, doi: 10.21037/apm.2017.06.23.

Dr. Kluger says that prior to the Summit, the leading neurology textbooks had not covered topics related to patient terminal care preferences or requests to end life. The conference has since been followed by publication of two handbooks on neuropalliative care, and these topics are now beginning to be better addressed.[12,13] There have also been two annual meetings of the International Neuropalliative Care Society, which is not only global and interdisciplinary but also *person-centered*. This refers to its practice of inviting people and their families who are living with these disorders to participate in the Society's events.[14]

Reminiscent of the literature on breaking bad news,[15] which has long been available to educate clinicians on how to impart unfortunate prognostic information in a sensitive and effective manner, there is a list of useful phrases to facilitate conversation with patients—like Dan—who say they wish to hasten death.[16] Clinician-educators have also enumerated potential barriers that are likely to hinder meaningful communication with patients. They have distinguished between different stages in patient decision-making processes, including a *pre-contemplative phase* when the person is wondering about options and gathering information about how to end life, a *contemplation phase* when the individual is considering hastening death but has not committed to a course of action, and a *determination phase*, in which people have decided—like Dan—that they want to pursue the provision of accelerated dying.

In addition to neurologists, the other medical specialists with expertise in managing problems of people with cognitive disorders are geriatric psychiatrists and especially geriatricians, like Dr. Bonasera. However, there are a relatively miniscule number of them in North America.[17] A Canadian report from 2020 stated that there are only 327 geriatricians in a country with 7 million citizens

---

[12] Neal Weisbrod and Timothy E. Quill, "Addressing and managing requests to hasten death," in Claire Creutzfeldt, Benzi Kluger and Robert Holloway (eds.), *Neuropalliative Care* (Cham: Springer, 2019), https://doi.org/10.1007/978-3-319-93215-6_14.

[13] Janis M. Miyasaki and Benzi M. Kluger (eds.), *Neuropalliative Care: Part I* (New York: Elsevier, 2022).

[14] INPCS, accessed December 29, 2022, https://www.inpcs.org/i4a/pages/index.cfm?pageid=3273.

[15] R. Buckman, "Breaking bad news: Why is it still so difficult?," *British Medical Journal (Clinical Research Edition)* 288, no. 6430 (May 1984): 1597–1599, doi: 10.1136/bmj.288.6430.1597.

[16] Aynharan Sinnaragjah, Andrea Feldstain, and Eric Wasylenko, "Responding to requests for hastened death in patients living with advanced neurologic disease," *Handbook of Clinical Neurology* 190 (2022): 217–237, in Janis M. Miyasaki and Benzi M. Kluger (eds.), *Neuropalliative Care: Part I* (New York: Elsevier B.V.A., 2022), https://doi.org/10.1016/B978-0-323-85029-2.00002-6.

[17] "Neurologist demographics and statistics in the US," Zippia, accessed October 22, 2022, https://www.zippia.com/neurologist-jobs/demographics/.

older than 65; this translates into 1 geriatrician for every 20,905 seniors.[18] The United States has only slightly better numbers, with 8,220 full-time practicing geriatricians, an older adult population of 52 million people, and a ratio of 1 geriatrician to 6,375 patients.[19] Twenty U.S. states have been labeled "dementia neurology deserts," as they are projected to have fewer than 10 neurologists per 10,000 people with dementia in 2025.[20]

In 2020, there were approximately 47,000 family medicine and general practice physicians across Canada,[21] while 2018 estimates in the United States find approximately 105,000 full-time equivalent family physicians and 82,000 general internal physicians (as well as 64,000 nurse clinicians and 33,000 full-time equivalent physician assistants) in primary care.[22]

According to geriatrician and palliative medicine practitioner Dr. Maura Brennan (email of January 26, 2023): "Honestly, the issue is not really whether the person living with dementia and the family are seen by neurology, geriatric psychiatry, primary care, or geriatrics. What patients really need is someone with expertise in the disease who can walk with them through the trajectory of the illness. Neither is neuropalliative care *the* answer. Many physicians trained in palliative medicine and neurology lack expertise in core geriatrics principles around evaluating and managing problems which commonly arise as dementia progresses—some examples include agitation from fear or suffering, delirium (hallucinations or abrupt confusion from medical problems),[23,24] side effects from drugs that should be dose adjusted or avoided in older people, and fall

---

[18] Megan DeLaire, "Canada not equipped to handle rising rates of dementia: Report," *CTVNews*, accessed October 20, 2022, https://www.ctvnews.ca/health/canada-not-equipped-to-handle-rising-rates-of-dementia-report-1.6115928.

[19] "Geriatrics workforce by the numbers," American Geriatric Society, accessed October 22, 2022, https://www.americangeriatrics.org/geriatrics-profession/about-geriatrics/geriatrics-workforce-numbers.

[20] "Alzheimer's disease facts and figures," Alzheimer's Association, accessed April 17, 2023, https://www.alz.org/alzheimers-dementia/facts-figures?utm_source=google&utm_medium=paidsearch&utm_campaign=google_grants&utm_content=alzheimers&gad=1&gclid=EAIaIQobChMIts_OucCu_gIVwejjBx3OGgx0EAAYASAAEgI1x_D_BwE.

[21] Frédéric Michas, "Number of Canadian family and general practitioners 2020, by province," Statista, accessed January 23, 2023, https://www.statista.com/statistics/831118/canada-family-general-practitioners-by-province/.

[22] "Primary care workforce projections," HRSA Health Workforce, accessed January 23, 2023, https://bhw.hrsa.gov/data-research/projecting-health-workforce-supply-demand/primary-health.

[23] Sharon K. Inouye, Rudi G. J. Westendorp, and Jane S. Saczynski, "Delirium in elderly people," *Lancet* 383, no. 9920 (March 2014): 911–922, doi: 10.1016/S0140-6736(13)60688-1.

[24] Sabha Ganai, K. Francis Lee, Andrea Merrill, et al., "Adverse outcomes of geriatric patients undergoing abdominal surgery who are at high risk for delirium," *Archives of Surgery* 142, no. 11 (November 2007): 1072–1078, doi: 10.1001/archsurg.142.11.1072.

reduction strategies.[25] One could say the same thing for geriatricians—that they may have gaps in managing drugs at the end of life in order to optimize symptom control, and they may be uncertain as to when to refer to hospice.[26,27] In short, we each have limitations, this system is desperately fragmented, and every clinician is pressed for time."

"What these patients really require," according to Dr. Brennan, a professor in the Department of Medicine at the University of Massachusetts Chan Medical School-Baystate, "is a *team* more than a *specific type of doctor*. They need social work to assist with the complicated shifts in family dynamics and interpersonal relationships as their abilities decline. They need spiritual support to blunt the suffering of the existential threat. They need a community health worker to educate and link them to appropriate services and resources. They need physician assistants or nurse practitioners and registered nurses to track symptoms, assess shifting challenges, and enlist colleagues over time. Some of the best evidence of improved outcomes for people with dementia is not a result of drugs or difficult medical decision-making. Coaching and support for caregivers often has the greatest impact. Many of these programs are designed by occupational therapists."[28]

As far as I know, like most patients, Dan lacked access to such a team, and this may have been considerably more important that the presence or absence of a neurologist.

And why didn't he have the resource of a team? Why are these so uncommon?

Again, I am indebted to Dr. Brennan, who points out that there are multiple contributing factors, including workforce issues, ageism, knowledge gaps, economics, and therapeutic nihilism, among others. However, her most succinct answer is that our medical system is simply not structured to support and pay for the team-based care which most older people need and deserve.

[25] Munther Queisi, Suheil Albert Atallah-Yunes, Farah Adamali, et al., "Frailty recognition by clinicians and its impact on advance care planning," *American Journal of Hospice and Palliative Care* 38, no. 4 (April 2021): 371–375, doi: 10.1177/1049909121995603.

[26] John R. F. Gladman, Simon Paul Conroy, Anette Hylen Ranhoff, and Adam Lee Gordon, "New horizons in the implementation and research of comprehensive geriatric assessment: Knowing, doing and the 'know-do' gap," *Age & Ageing* 45, no. 2 (March 2016): 194–200, doi: 10.1093/ageing. afw012.

[27] Claire E. Magauran and Maura J. Brennan, "Patient-doctor communication and the importance of clarifying end-of-life decisions," *American Journal of Hospice and Palliative Care* 22, no. 5 (September-October 2005): 335–336, doi: 10.1177/104990910502200504.

[28] Sally Bennett, Kate Laver, Sebastian Voigt-Radloff, et al., "Occupational therapy for people with dementia and their family carers provided at home: A systematic review and meta-analysis," *BMJ Open* 9, no. 11 (November 2019):e026308, doi: 10.1136/bmjopen-2018-026308.

Dan would have been the first person to clear his throat and gently suggest that he wasn't like most people diagnosed with dementias—he was young, male, physically fit, educated, and fortunate in still retaining his ability to reason and communicate. In addition, he had multiple contacts within the medical establishment, ample financial resources, a supportive spouse, and a large friendship and kinship network.

All true!

But even Dan could have reaped benefits from a team approach—especially if it would have been respectful of his wish to control the timing and means of dying. And the systemic shortcoming that he faced is not limited to the United States but is a global Alzheimer's problem.[29] Healthcare for people with dementia should ideally be continuous, holistic, and integrated across providers. Instead, current healthcare systems are fractured, uncoordinated, and unresponsive to the needs of patients and their families.[30,31,32,33,34] In high-income nations, they tend to be highly specialized from the point of diagnosis onward, with little appreciation of coordinated primary care services.

Little has changed since the 2016 World Alzheimer Report stated "Dementia is currently under-detected, underdiagnosed, under-disclosed, under-treated

[29] M. Prince, A. Comas-Herrera, and M. Knapp, "World Alzheimer report 2016: Improving healthcare for people living with dementia: Coverage, quality and costs now and in the future," Alzheimer's Disease International, 2016, https://www.alzint.org/resource/world-alzheimer-report-2016

[30] Jane Lowers, Melissa Scardaville, Sean Hughes, and Nancy J. Preston, "Comparison of the experience of caregiving at end of life or in hastened death: A narrative synthesis review," *BMC Palliative Care* 19, no. 154 (October 2020), https//doi.org/10.1186/s12904-02-00660-8.

[31] Sheila Holmes, Ellen Wiebe, Jessica Shaw, et al., "Exploring the experience of supporting a loved one through a medically assisted death in Canada," *Canadian Family Physician* 64, no. 9 (September 2018): e387–e393, PMID: 30209112, PMCID: PMC6135137.

[32] Nikkie B. Swarte, Marije L. van de Lee, Johanna G. van der Bom, et al., "Effects of euthanasia on the bereaved families and friends: A cross sectional study," *British Medical Journal* 327, no. 7408 (July 2003): 189, doi: 10.1136/bmj.327.7408.189.

[33] Claudia Gamondi, Murielle Pott, Karen Forbesand, and Sheila Payne, "Exploring the experiences of bereaved families involved in assisted suicide in Southern Switzerland: A qualitative study," *BMJ Supportive & Palliative Care* 5, no. 2 (June 2015): 146–152, doi: 10.1136/bmjspcare-2013000483.

[34] Linda Ganzini, Elizabeth R. Goy, Steven K. Dobscha, and Holly Prigerson, "Mental health outcomes of family members of Oregonians who request physician aid in dying," *Journal of Pain and Symptom Management* 38, no. 6 (December 2009): 807–815, doi: 10.1016/j.jpainsymman.2009.04.026.

and under-managed in primary care."[35] The document specifically noted: "There is also a policy gap regarding end-of-life care for people with dementia. The focus is on living well with dementia, with relatively less attention to the complex medical, social, and ethical management of the physical decline that leads to death."

[35] "Prince et al., "World Alzheimer report 2016.".

21

If Dan had been eligible for medical assistance in dying (MAiD), he would have likely also arranged to be a transplant donor, as is possible in Belgium, the Netherlands, Spain, and Canada.[1,2] But John and he knew his organs couldn't be salvaged following the proposed overdose, and, many months earlier, the two men had instead contacted Oregon Health and Science University (OHSU) to discuss donating his cadaver. Now, they decided it was time to reconnect with OHSU and further clarify what the process entailed. John was in his art studio several blocks away when he placed the call. During the conversation, John asked the program's manager if it would make any difference whether the death followed an intentional overdose, and she replied, "No."

However, about 3 minutes later, John's cellphone rang. He told me, "It was the same woman saying, 'Because you mentioned suicide, I'm legally required to notify the police. I'm sorry to have to do this, but I don't have a choice. Very shortly, they will be showing up at the condominium.'"

"She had already made the call to the authorities?" I asked.

"Yup," said John, "and she apologized to me. I detected no malice on her part and completely understood the position she was in. I felt like it was institutionally the right thing for her to do."

"What happened next?" I inquired.

"I hung up and immediately called Dan to let him know what was occurring."

[1] Kim Wiebe, Lindsay C. Wilson, Ken Lotherington, Caitlin Mills, Sam D. Shemie, and James Downar, "Deceased organ and tissue donation after medical assistance in dying: 2023 updated guidance for policy," *CMAJ* 195, no. 25 (June 2023): E870–E878, https://doi.org/10.1503/cmaj.230108.

[2] Johannes Mulder, Hans Sonneveld, Dirk Van Raemdonck, et al., "Practice and challenges for organ donation after medical assistance in dying: A scoping review including the results of the first international roundtable in 2021," *American Journal of Transplantation* 22, no. 12 (December 2022): 2759–2780, doi: 10.1111/ajt.17198.

"Was this a 'Holy shit, I can't believe it' sort of moment?"

"Well," he said. "I'm aware that time is usually of the essence when it comes to people who are despairing and going to commit suicide. On some level, the woman knew that wasn't our situation, and she was contrite. But at the same time—and I don't want to overstate it—yes, I was shocked."

"Shocked?"

"About the reality of what we were doing—that Dan was going to take his life, and the shit had just hit the fan." But one's psychological defenses kick in and John explained, "At the same time, we were both just very matter of fact with the knowledge that the police would be showing up. Dan did not freak out. I didn't freak out. Even though it was the first example of how things can go wrong. It seems strange now, but we didn't completely freak out."

"And what happened next?"

"I was still several blocks away at the studio when two police officers knocked on the apartment door. They stood at the threshold and began talking to Dan. He told me later that one of them was a man, one was a woman, they were both quite young—in their 30s—and each was in a uniform, carrying a firearm, and wearing a protective mask."

Dan explained to John that the police officers' body language, tone of voice, and the words they chose to use all combined to be calming. Certainly, neither of them was jangling handcuffs or making any kind of threats. They were merely asking questions and exploring the situation. For Dan, it became another opportunity to tell his story, to recount the truth. He neither stammered nor acted self-defensively. The interaction ended with one of the police—the man—tearfully describing to Dan the consequences of his grandmother's Alzheimer's on the family. For 20, 30, or 40minutes—Dan had trouble estimating time—the three of them quietly spoke to each other. They conversed as human being to human being to human being.

According to John, "At the conclusion, the two officers reassured Dan: 'We're not going to pursue this anymore. We understand what your situation is.' Before departing, they wished him well on his journey, and, if this interaction hadn't taken place during the pandemic, they would undoubtably have hugged him or at the very least shaken his hand."

"My God," I exclaimed.

"Can you make this stuff up, Lew?" John asked.

"Definitely not," I replied.

"It was beautiful in a certain way," said John. "They were well trained, and they stripped away the anxiety. Dan got to tell them his truth, and they responded with theirs. It is remarkable that what could have been a terrible institutional experience was transformed into a deeply personal one."

Dan would explain to me at our next interview that his immediate reaction to the visit by the police officers was to feel "triumphant." It left him more certain than ever that the plan to end his life was justified.

*****

According to John, despite the flurry of back-and-forth calls with Dan's inner circle of loved ones and notwithstanding the visit by the police, "Neither of us really seriously considered that anything would go wrong."

Which is why they were dumbfounded when a couple of days later, one of the Winter family apparently telephoned Portland's suicide prevention hotline.

That same afternoon there was a knock on the condominium door, which is very rare because one normally must electronically unlock the main entrance to first let people into the building. Both men glanced at each other to see if they were expecting any visitors, and they then assumed it must be one of their neighbors paying a rare visit. Instead, when John opened the door, he discovered two complete strangers. They were a couple dressed like stereotypical Portland hipsters: he had a man-bun hairstyle, she a knitted cap of variegated colored yarn, and both wore puffy winter coats and jeans. Like the police officers who appeared earlier, the two of them were in their mid to late 30s and projected youthful optimism and energy.

According to John, "They asked to come in. I automatically said, 'No.' I was really shaken to realize that our home was being invaded yet again."

Dan heard them beginning to introduce themselves, and he walked over and stood alongside his husband. The four of them were positioned 6 feet apart at the doorway and each donned surgical masks. The young couple were calm, and their language was colloquial and jargon-free, but also deadly serious. They had come from the Multnomah County Suicide Prevention Office after an anonymous call alerted them that a person in the household was considering ending life.

Dan proceeded to confidently describe exactly what he intended to do and why.

John said, "The young couple's demeanor led both of us to trust them. They were completely nonconfrontational and well suited for what they were doing. I felt very reassured, and I also knew we were not the typical people they were used to meeting. They were accustomed to dealing with anguish, anger, and conflict, and God knows what. . . ."

I suggested, "Substance abuse?"

"Yeah," he replied, "that, too. . . . But instead, they were facing two exceedingly composed and reasonable adults who seemed to be very much in control of their own lives."

"We talked with the couple from the Suicide Response Team for nearly half an hour," John said. "It was a very thorough conversation. Before departing, like the police officers, they also wished Dan well on his journey."

But that same evening, the landline phone rang, and it was yet another young person, who introduced himself as an employee of the Multnomah County Adult Protective Services. He, too, had been notified that someone in the household was considering suicide.

When I heard about his call, I immediately assumed that concerns were raised by the Winter family about whether John represented a threat to Dan's safety.

The man said, "I'm sorry, but there is a series of questions I'm required to ask."

Dan began by telling him, "I'm not going to comment on the motivations of my family member for making this referral to you, but I'm a 62-year-old, otherwise healthy guy. I've still got a pretty decent hold on my cognitive ability."

The phone was put on speaker and a three-way conversation ensued over the next hour and a half. "Yup," John said, "we talked for 90 minutes!" By the conclusion, John reported, "We were chuckling a little bit with him, as he said, 'If there's ever anything that I can do for either of you, please call. Under any other circumstances, I would really like to get to know you guys better!'"

"It made us proud to be living in Portland," said John, "where liberal values have encouraged institutions that can very easily go in the direction of confrontation and negativity—the police, suicide squad, and protective services—to instead engage in really profound, meaningful interactions."

*****

A few days later, before calling John and Dan, I had been listening to a dissonant piece of Stravinsky's music on the radio. Hardly my favorite composer, I frequently had difficulty enjoying his unusual harmonies, understanding his orchestrations, or grasping his rhythmic energy. But it proved to be an apt selection because, as they picked up the telephone, I found that the two men were no longer in the same emotional place as before. With the passage of time, they had begun to feel increasingly incensed with the individual or individuals from the family who had set into motion "the insulting wellness checks." The couple was no longer satisfied with the outcome of the visits and the telephone calls. Rather, they were now thoroughly alarmed and fearful at how things were spinning out of control.

"For the first time in this whole process," John said, "we are afraid of what might happen to Dan and me. We have never previously locked the door to our condominium. But now, before we take Friday for a walk, we carefully look out the glass doors and scan the cars across the street. We don't immediately leave the building before checking. We try to spot any official Portland or Multnomah County vehicles and to ascertain whether anyone might be waiting for us to appear. We have never been paranoid previously, but we are suddenly very, very paranoid."

The couple explained they were worried that a family member might be arranging to commit Dan to a psychiatric facility or get him declared mentally incompetent or have a guardian or conservator appointed. This did not strike me as being completely loony, as I had previously written about an elderly physician, Dr. David Raff, who was committed to a Florida psychiatric hospital for the first time in his life when authorities were informed that he was helping his wife, Reba, who had a mild dementing illness, to acquire medications for an overdose.[3]

Discharged a couple of days later because of the active intervention of his two adult sons—both of whom were also physicians—David and Reba Raff purposefully resumed their peaceful lives for the next month, carried on with their usual routines, and stopped talking about either her Alzheimer's or about dying. Then, when things had calmed down, with the full cooperation and support of their family, the couple quietly overdosed together.

Back in Portland, Dan heard rumors and began to doubt whether he'd be able to extricate himself from the tightening coils of Alzheimer's and the wishes of certain family members to prolong his life. He was terrified that his rights could suddenly be abrogated.

Who is going to question us next? he mused. *Are we going to be interrogated by the National Guard? Homeland Security? Perhaps the ASPCA?* Dan hadn't entirely lost his sense of humor, but he had slipped into a surreal nightmare with Monty Pythonesque aspects.

As I listened, my own imagination shifted into high gear. I know it's melodramatic, but I couldn't help but think again about the Winter ancestors and of "Bleeding Kansas." I heard ghostlike horses neighing in the night, the crack of Minié balls fired from distant muskets, neighbors arguing with neighbors about slavery, and furious threats of violence and mayhem. I knew that in the present day, directly beneath Dan and John's windows, were genuine rioters racing through the streets of Portland. Motivated by individual precepts of patriotism or social justice, the mob's rowdiness was documented almost every night on national news broadcasts. Enraged people were stirred up by the pandemic, its dangers and frustrations—including otherwise peaceable citizens who punched airplane flight attendants or screamed at supermarket managers

[3] Lewis M. Cohen, *A Dignified Ending: Taking Control Over How We Die* (Lanham, MD: Rowman & Littlefield, 2019), 15–19, 53–61.

and even shot and killed a security guard at a Dollar store for trying to enforce mask regulations.[4] From Dan's perspective, the present-day Winter clan was a volatile mix: politically connected, well-versed in the law, with their roots firmly immersed in the Catholic Church and the Rockefeller wing of the Republican Party. It didn't seem impossible to conceive of a kidnapping or a civil suit intended to forestall his death. It wasn't out of the question that John might face criminal accusations and repercussions.

And then I asked myself, *Is it paranoid when the things that you fear may realistically occur? Especially, when they have taken place with others in similar situations.*

I remembered listening to author Katie Engelhart's description of an elderly, retired Oxford-educated professor whose door was literally broken down by police the night before she was to take her life with a Nembutal overdose.[5] She had been quite open about the plan with friends, physicians, and acquaintances in her small village in southwest England, and she had joined a global right-to-die organization called Exit International, whose members hailed from the United Kingdom, Canada, America, Australia, and New Zealand. The woman turned out to be one of several people from the group who were identified and targeted by Interpol. No doubt the law enforcement authorities in each of these countries felt justified in trying to prevent them from killing themselves, but. . . .

And I remembered writing in considerable detail about the legal problems of the Final Exit Network (FEN), a right-to-die organization that underwent three separate court cases after having become the object of an elaborate undercover sting by the Georgia Bureau of Investigation (GBI).[6] The GBI probed whether FEN volunteers had crossed a legal line and were guilty of assisting suicides. Each of the court cases was triggered by family members who hadn't been told by the individuals who died that they intended to hasten their deaths—mainly because it was doubtful that their loved ones would have accepted them going ahead. Faye Girsh, a right-to-die activist and founder of the Hemlock Society of San Diego, wrote me (March 7, 2023, interview), "We used to refer to clients like those as 'prisoners of the family.' "

During the investigation, the GBI uncovered and then circulated a lengthy list of people who sought or were seeking membership in FEN. This, too, led to a series of "wellness checks" around the United States, which mainly consisted

---

[4] Livia Albeck-Ripka, "3 relatives get life in prison for killing security guard over mask dispute," *The New York Times*, accessed January 22, 2023, https://www.nytimes.com/2023/01/20/us/michigan-family-dollar-shooting-sentence.html.

[5] Terry Gross, "Inside the fight for the right to die: Logistical and ethical challenges," NPR, Fresh Air, accessed October 1, 2022, https://www.npr.org/sections/health-shots/2021/03/09/975175847/inside-the-fight-for-the-right-to-die-logistical-and-ethical-challenges.

[6] Cohen, *A Dignified Ending*, 205–228.

of telephone calls and polite visits by local police rather than full-fledged-break-the-door-down raids, such as what had happened with Engelhart's professor.

I pictured Dan and John standing on the edge of a crumbling precipice—fearfully clutching each other while being buffeted by wind gusts. The two men always knew that theoretically they might lose control, and they had done everything conceivable to avoid such a situation (other than to keep the plan secret). But a storm was raging, and I felt ineffably sad.

I was originally convinced that, by being frank and honest, Dan had properly set the stage for his death. He was not engaged in an irrational or impulsive act to end life. He was genuinely tortured by a worsening condition and intractable suffering.

The columnist Jane E. Brody has written about the latter, "Intractable suffering is defined by patients, not doctors. . . . It's less a question of uncontrollable physical pain, which prompts only a minority of requests for medical aid in dying, than it is a loss of autonomy, a loss of dignity, a loss of quality of life and an inability to engage in what makes people's lives meaningful."[7]

John had carefully observed how Dan was steadily losing parts of himself, his identity, his personhood. The tall Kansan had carefully assembled the necessary ingredients to achieve a peaceful demise at a time of his own choosing. And this process included vigorously attempting to marshal the support of his entire extended family. To learn that some of his beloved kinfolk now threatened and challenged him was for me a moment of great perplexity.

But the calamitous consequences of speaking freely about his plans to die was not puzzling to legal authority Susan Stefan, JD, who explained (December 8, 2022, interview): "It is vitally important that individuals who are considering ending their lives be able to talk freely. However, there are so many structural disincentives, people generally end up being unable to communicate about this crucially important decision, because they—realistically—are unsure who they can trust." She went on to comment that "Even when the figures of authority are as respectful and empathic as the police, suicide prevention, and adult protective services people who Dan encountered (which is quite rare), the very power they represent can be scary and intimidating. It is tragic, but society undermines its own goals of suicide prevention."[8]

[7] Jane E. Brody, "When patients choose to end their lives: For some, the decision to die is more complicated than a wish to reduce pain," *The New York Times*, accessed May 18, 2023, https://www.nytimes.com/2021/04/05/well/live/aid-in-dying.html.

[8] Rebecca Dresser, "Dementia, disability, and advance medical directives: Defensible standards for dementia care," in *Disability, Health, Law, and Bioethics*, ed. I. Glenn Cohen (Cambridge University Press, 2020), 77–88, doi:10.1017/9781108622851.010.

I asked Stefan to expound on her last sentence, and she replied: "The predominant emotion or mindset reported by Dr. Edwin Shneidman, the father of suicidology, was being 'stuck'—not seeing any way out of their current life/problems. People also report feeling very isolated and alone. If people were able to freely discuss their suicidality, without the situation being immediately escalated to involuntary detention and hospitalization, they might both feel less alone and actually obtain some insight/solution/comfort to the problems that seem so overwhelming."

I considered Dan to be a courageous and forthright individual. Granted, I did not know him during the earlier period when he was admittedly deceitful and led a double life. But since then, he earnestly endeavored to be different and more authentic. He not only confronted and overcame a host of tribulations and maladaptive behaviors, but he had tirelessly invested himself in reestablishing loving connections with his impressively large network of friends and kin as well as achieving a successful, decade-long marriage to John. If he was now—at least in my imagination—metaphorically standing on the edge of the cliff, then what did it herald for anyone else who tried to follow his path?

22

I connected with Dan for our next scheduled interview on January 6, 2021. I had just begun my standard consent request for his permission to record our conversation when John entered the room. I heard him explain to Dan that Congress was being invaded by a mob of protestors from the President's rally. He was watching on television as demonstrators fought with police inside and outside of the Capitol halls, angrily flailing about with flags, iron bars, and plastic riot shields. Crowds flowed into the building's entrances amid clouds of chemical irritants, flash-bangs, and overturned barricades. The ferocious scuffles, bloodshed, shouting, and singing of "The Star-Spangled Banner" evoked for me the etchings I have seen of the storming of the Bastille, which had taken place along similar lines some 230 years earlier.

It took me about 2 seconds to realize that this was an inopportune time to conduct an interview, and we rescheduled for the following day.

When I called back, Dan's first words were, "I'm having a tough time." But he was not talking about the insurrection in Washington.

"Oh?"

"There's been a lot of drama, which, Jesus Christ on a crutch, is really getting to me. I feel like I'm making all kinds of mistakes, and I've been trying to keep myself busy by conversing with people."

He had been hearing more whispers that family members were considering initiating guardianship or conservatorship proceedings—legal arrangements typically reserved as a last resort to assume control over severely incapacitated, vulnerable people. There are an estimated 1.3 million conservatorships in the United States.[1] Yes, that's *million*. While nowadays most Americans are cognizant

---

[1] Dennis Thompson, "How 1.3 million Americans became controlled by conservatorships," *U.S. News & World Report*, accessed October 2, 2022, https://www.usnews.com/news/health-news/articles/2021-10-18/how-13-million-americans-became-controlled-by-conservatorships#:~:text=About%201.3%20million%20guardianship%20or,the%20National%20Council%20on%20Disability.

of Britney Spears's legal struggles with her father, they are less aware of situations that have involved other celebrities, including the singer Joni Mitchell, the performer and composer Brian Wilson of the Beachboys, and the actor Mickey Rooney, who were each troubled by mental health problems and placed under conservatorship.

For Dan, this development would have been the worst possible scenario that he and John could imagine happening. They felt like their world was descending into total chaos.

Dan initiated a flurry of phone calls to friends and family. He told me, "A couple of individuals said, 'I can't support you. I don't agree with your plan. I think that what you're doing is selfish and cruel to your elderly mother and your children.'"

This made him think, *Everybody used to be uniformly supportive. But when it became a real thing . . . suddenly there was anger and fear and tears.*

Under the emotional strain, Dan's Alzheimer's symptoms worsened. "I forget who I'm talking with," he complained. "I forget what time my appointments are. I'm messing up everything, from going to the supermarket, to trying to cook something, to taking out the dog. Nothing is going right. My attention span is so much shorter . . . and the most fearsome and arguably gruesome symptom is not knowing where the fuck you are—especially when you're in a familiar place."

His voice got louder as he described waking up and having a terrible time trying to figure out what to put on—how to get dressed. "The clean jeans and the flannel shirt that I wear almost every day were right in front of me. I was looking at them thinking, *That's not appropriate. . . .* Lew, weird shit is happening. . . . I'm failing to remember big chunks of how to live."

Dan began questioning whether he ought to not leave the house by himself, and how that would be "a significant loss of agency." He feared that he could no longer take Friday for her walks.

I commented to him that his Alzheimer's, "Certainly ain't a barrel of monkeys," and he countered with, "Dementia is more like a murder of crows." Lacking familiarity with the expression, I had to look it up and learned that it is based on an ancient superstitious belief that flocks of birds would peck out the eyes of corpses abandoned in heaps on battlefields. Dan's metaphor evoked for me the monstrous images which Hieronymus Bosch painted 500 years ago.

Dan decided that when they had announced the date for his impending death, "It was just too soon for some of the Winter clan emotionally." After considering what to do about it, he and John had just finished composing an email to inform the entire family that Dan was *not* going to die on January 15. He would also *not* employ lethal medications. The email tried to make it clear that Dan desperately needed some peace and solitude to better consider his situation. The couple hoped these measures might quell the family's tumult. John and Dan wanted some time to regroup and think things over together.

I seriously wondered whether Dan's plan to end his life was irreparably shattered. He sounded distraught, and his thinking was more disorganized. I worried that he had not only misjudged the reaction of the Winters but had delayed too long—that midnight had arrived and Cinderella's gown had transformed back into rags. She forlornly stood outside the ballroom surrounded by scampering rodents and a solitary pumpkin.

*****

However, when we spoke several days later, things had changed. Dan now sounded considerably more composed. "The other night," he reported, "John and I had a really good videoconference call with Barbara Coombs Lee, the founder of Compassion & Choices (C&C), along with the organization's legal director, who is an old friend of mine." Lee empathized with the couple's distress and their fear that the family might try to intervene legally. She had not apparently endorsed the original plan to overdose and was pleased that Dan had announced his decision to abandon this method. During the call, a question was raised as to whether he might instead reconsider voluntarily stopping eating and drinking (VSED) as an option.[2]

According to Timothy Kirk, a bioethics researcher, "[VSED] is probably the lowest-tech, oldest form of hastening your death."[3] He continued, "Some people would probably look at this as a form of suicide. I don't, because for me suicide is connected to disordered thinking, to impairment, often psychiatric, but not always."

VSED, Kirk explained, requires substantial resolve on the part of the individual and their loved ones, as well as, ideally, a cooperative medical and nursing team. Depending on the health of the patient, it may take up to a month before death ensues. But—and this is crucial—VSED is legally permissible in jurisdictions where medical aid in dying is not. It is also not restricted to people with terminal illnesses. Furthermore, it is an accepted way to die in Hinduism

---

[2] Robin Marantz Henig, "If you have dementia, can you hasten death as you wished?," NPR, All Things Considered, accessed January 20, 2023, https://www.npr.org/sections/health-shots/2015/02/10/382725729/if-you-have-dementia-can-you-hasten-death-as-you-wished.

[3] Laurie Loisel, "Decision by Lee Hawkins to stop eating and drinking prompts new policy at VNA & Hospice of Cooley Dickinson," *Daily Hampshire Gazette*, September 23, 2014, https://www.gazettenet.com/Archives/2014/09/VSEDpolicyhawkinsside-hg-092414.

and Jainism by persons who are terminally ill, suffering from great disability, have no desire or ambition left, or no responsibilities remaining in life.[4,5]

Although Dan had described to me some months earlier why he originally rejected this method to accelerate his death, that was *then* and this was *now*. In the beginning of his deliberations, "an overdose seemed easier," he clarified. But at the present time, "I'm over the worry about stopping eating and drinking being horrible. I think it will actually give some of my loved ones the opportunity to say that he didn't kill himself."

"Do you have any reason to believe your family is going to react differently if it's VSED and not an overdose?" I asked.

"That's a good question," he replied. "I don't expect them to be exactly comfortable with VSED. . . . But I'm oddly comforted, because knowing my family, I think there will be people who would prefer to say he died of natural causes. Those individuals might consider dehydration to be a more 'natural cause.' "

I inquired about the importance of the social stigma of suicide, and he responded, "There are a couple in the crew who still identify as Catholic, and there's no key to heaven for people who suicide." He went on to say that VSED, again, might be more acceptable to them.

Sounding hopeful, Dan finished, "In the meantime, I've changed how I want to die. I can't really tell you why I like that better than going all out in one instant." His voice then rose in pitch, and he began repeating, "I don't know. I don't know. Hell, I don't know."

Barbara Coombs Lee, who was trained as a family nurse practitioner, a physician assistant, and a lawyer—and who went on to found C&C—affirmed (August 31, 2021, interview) that in her opinion, "Dan is in his right mind. He is perfectly decisionally capable and any effort to thwart [his decision to stop eating and drinking] will be a violation of his right to privacy."

When I asked her about C&C, she said, "We see it as our role to remove the legal and societal barriers, and to remove the taboo."

During her conversation with Dan, she suggested that John would be less likely to face even the miniscule possibility of an assisted-suicide criminal accusation if they employed what bioethicist Paul Menzel and others call, "preemptive VSED."[6] Menzel, Professor of Philosophy Emeritus at Pacific Lutheran

---

[4] "Right to die," Wikipedia, accessed August 20, 2022, https://en.wikipedia.org/wiki/Right_to_die#India.

[5] "Prayopavesa," Wikipedia, accessed August 20, 2022, https://en.wikipedia.org/wiki/Prayopavesa.

[6] Dena Davis and Paul T. Metzel, "Ethical issues," in *Voluntarily Stopping Eating and Drinking: A Compassionate, Widely Available Option for Hastening Death*, eds. Timothy E. Quill, Paul T. Menzel, Thaddeus M. Pope, and Judith K. Schwarz (New York: Oxford University Press, 2021), 197–198.

University, defines this (June 10, 2023, email) as being a subcategory of VSED that is undertaken by a patient not because they necessarily regard their current suffering or prolonged dying as intolerable, but because they don't want to miss the opportunity by losing decision-making capacity. The person is willing to forego some life they regard as worth living to avoid an unacceptable quality of life in the future. This course of action is likely be satisfactory to local hospices, which can offer the benefits of acute symptom management and bereavement care.

Dan conferred with the C&C attorney who agreed to act as his "shield," and the lawyer reassured the couple that he would ward off any attempts by family members to assume guardianship or conservatorship. According to Dan: "The man said that there's nothing illegal if you're going to kill yourself by not eating and drinking. Nobody's going to come to your door. . . . You have a right not to be harassed about this. You have a right to privacy."

23

Dan next reached out to Eric Walsh, MD, a retired, local palliative medicine physician who, he observed is, "one of those people with a special gift for communicating. Furthermore, he's very generous with himself, his information, and opinions." Dan and John were struck by the man's decency. They spoke several times about voluntarily stopping eating and drinking (VSED) and whether Portland hospices would offer symptom management. Dr. Walsh had been consulted when Brittany Maynard made use of the state's death-with-dignity law, and he also helped between 15 and 20 patients die through VSED. He agreed to informally consult with Dan but would not be managing his care. With Dan's consent, Dr. Walsh, Emeritus Professor of Family Medicine and Emeritus Professor of Internal Medicine at Oregon Health and Science University, and I also discussed the situation.

The palliative care clinician clarified (October 8, 2021, interview) that technically the diagnosis of Alzheimer's alone was insufficient to qualify Dan for hospice. According to the regulations, the disease would need to have progressed to the point of bowel and bladder incontinence and an inability on the patient's part to speak more than six words in a single day.

However, in his opinion, hospices should automatically provide services to people undergoing VSED. But hospices are unfortunately not doing this because of a "culture of anxiety about being investigated." He explained to me that the federal government commissioned private companies to oversee all hospice charges, and these companies only receive payment when they uncover "fraud and abuse." Dr. Walsh went on to say that "this perverse incentive" prompts hospice staff and medical directors to be very conservative about admitting people into hospice care because they fear being financially penalized. Most hospices run on exceedingly tight budgets; they can ill afford to be accused of not following the rules and then face the possibility of closure if forced to unexpectedly reimburse insurers.

In contrast to Dr. Walsh's generally sanguine opinion about the hospice industry, there are some who express concern that, since 2010, "the death business has been infiltrated by an onslaught of professional grifters."[1] A report by the Center for Economic and Policy Research finds that the care of the dying is now a $22.4 billion business, and an industry that began with mainly small, ethically sound, nonprofit providers is now dominated by for-profit hospices. Wall Street players, driven by the logic of profit maximization, are buying up the existing nonprofit agencies and consolidating them into large chains with hundreds of locations.[2] Regulations are inadequate and enforcement lax, which has provided opportunities for the flourishing of dishonest hospice facilities. The report concludes that, as a result, waste, abuse, and fraud are becoming widespread.

I asked Dr. Walsh: "Do you have any doubts about Dan's current capacity to make life and death decisions? What is his prognosis if he doesn't take an overdose or make use of VSED?"

The palliative medicine practitioner was confident that Dan still retained capacity and said, "If you consider the road between diagnosis and death in Alzheimer's disease to be 10 miles long, he's about 2 ½ miles into it. All of the truly awful stuff still lies ahead for him and John."

"How would you describe the 'awful stuff?'"

"Those last 7 ½ miles are some of the most hellish roads you could possibly tread as a human being—especially when one is in a loving relationship. You gradually disappear, and then stop caring that you're disappearing, and become really nothing but a burden."

"So, what do you tell people who are considering VSED?"

"My short version touches on three separate things. One is that many religious or spiritual practices endorse fasting, and . . . thirst and hunger last for a couple of days, and then they are usually replaced by a sense of elevated well-being.

"The second way of looking at VSED is that we are creatures on this green earth, just like dogs, horses, or elephants. Keep in mind that the natural response when animals near their end is to stop eating and drinking.

"The third point is that when someone refrains from eating and drinking, their body then produces ketones. If you've ever taken a long hike and didn't drink enough water and your urine looks really dark and smells funny, those are

[1] Maureen Tkacik, "Born to die: Medicare spends tens of billions of dollars on hospice care each year: A new report ponders why regulators insist on going easy on literal death merchants," The American Prospect, accessed May 11, 2023, https://prospect.org/health/2023-04-26-born-to-die-hospice-care/.

[2] Eileen Appelbaum, Rosemary Batt, and Emma Curchin, "Preying on the dying: Private equity gets rich in hospice care," CEPR, accessed May 10, 2023, https://cepr.net/report/preying-on-the-dying-private-equity-gets-rich-in-hospice-care/.

ketones. Ketones have a calming effect on the central nervous system. In fact, there are certain seizure disorders in childhood that can only be successfully treated with a ketogenic diet—a diet that promotes the formation of ketones."[3]

People more commonly hear about ketones in relation to diabetes. They are the chemicals produced when the body lacks insulin and begins to burn fat instead of glucose for energy; diabetics can slip into a metabolic state known as *ketoacidosis*.

"When people ask for additional details," the palliative medicine veteran continued, "I talk about a week of gradually diminishing awareness of the outside world and more of an internal focus. This is followed by around a week of unconsciousness, which usually does not appear to cause any untoward symptoms."

While I, too, felt buoyed up by Dr. Walsh's description, Robert K. Horowitz, MD, had some concerns that he expressed in an email (October 8, 2022). Dr. Horowitz is a contributing author to the recent textbook on VSED,[4] and the Gosnell Distinguished Professor in Palliative Care and Chief of Palliative Care Division at the University of Rochester Medical Center. He appreciated the thrust of Dr. Walsh's words but offered two challenges.

"The first," he explained, "is perhaps obvious but important: dying animals and gravely ill humans who are anorectic on the basis of their illness are very different from those who choose VSED, which by its design is *not* about the so-called 'nature of things.' Dying creatures (including humans) *can't* eat and drink." Yet, societal and family pressures compel us to feed seriously ill people *despite* the body (and maybe spirit) rejecting this. "VSED's 'voluntariness,'" he explained, "is precisely the opposite: it is a deliberate denial of the active drive to eat and drink. Dr. Walsh's words may be reassuring, but my strong sense is they are false, and I don't endorse them."

He went on to say, "If a family member offers this comparison, I do not feel compelled to challenge them—that would be unfair; but I do not believe we should offer this false comparison to reassure them."

Dr. Horowitz continued: "The second challenge is the paucity of evidence that fasting-induced ketosis causes euphoria—there were a few obesity/fasting observations in the 1950s, and some theoretical conjecture about this possibility in the early 2000s, but there is no convincing evidence this is reliably true." Studies have found that during the first few days to weeks of restrictive ketogenic

[3] Kirsty J. Martin-McGill, Cerian F. Jackson, Rebecca Bresnahan, Robert G. Levy, and Paul N. Cooper, "Ketogenic diets for drug-resistant epilepsy," *Cochrane Database of Systematic Reviews* 11, no. 11 (November 2018): CD001903, doi: 10.1002/14651858.CD001903.pub4.

[4] Dena Davis and Paul T. Metzel, "Ethical issues," in *Voluntarily Stopping Eating and Drinking: A Compassionate, Widely Available Option for Hastening Death*, eds. Timothy E. Quill, Paul T. Menzel, Thaddeus M. Pope, and Judith K. Schwarz (New York: Oxford University Press, 2021).

diets for epilepsy management, patients report fatigue, headache, nausea, constipation, hypoglycemia, and acidosis.[5]

Dr. Horowitz cautioned: "Here again is a potential disingenuous endorsement, or even persuasion, to wary patients and families. It *is* well demonstrated that what most people describe as hunger pangs diminish after a few days, but while I mention the possibility that they will feel at peace (due to any number of things *other* than ketones, e.g., relief, 'success', loving family presence and support, medications, etc.), I also [must acknowledge] that VSED is not uniformly peaceful—some people are moderately or very uncomfortable, agitated, and confused. [VSED is] not described by most who suffer or witness it as a pleasant, let alone a euphoric, experience. However, wonderfully, with meticulous, expert care, the presence of loved ones, and sometimes low, and sometimes escalating doses of medications, most people undergoing VSED can achieve ease."

Whether or not Dr. Walsh's words are disputed, they certainly offered much desired encouragement to Dan and John. The two men were especially buoyed to learn that he was confident the hospice affiliated with Dan's insurance carrier would provide services. The palliative medicine physician was less certain as to when those services would be instituted.

Dr. James A. Tulsky is Professor of Medicine at Harvard Medical School, and he has had a long-standing interest in doctor–patient communication and the quality of life in serious illnesses, especially congestive heart disease and cancer. What doesn't appear in his online biosketch is that he is also an observant Jew and a real mensch!

I was interested in his impression of Dr. Walsh's introduction to VSED, and I wasn't entirely surprised when he wrote (October 3, 2022): "The palliative care doctor's description that he gives his patients was troubling to me. I am personally not opposed to the practice, but it also feels like he may be trying to normalize something that isn't normal."

I asked Dr. Tulsky to address matters from an Orthodox Jewish perspective, and he commented: "To say in this context that 'many religious traditions endorse fasting,' would be wildly inappropriate for Judaism. As we enter Yom Kippur [he and I exchanged emails right before the Day of Atonement], fasting is indeed something that Jews are commanded to do six times a year. . . . *And*, there are strict rules that one is *not* obligated to fast if they are sick. Fasting is *not* supposed to lead to death, just to enhanced self-reflection. The Orthodox and some other Jewish denominations are definitely opposed to VSED."

---

[5] Lee Crosby, Brenda Davis, Shivam Joshi, Meghan Jardine, Jennifer Paul, Maggie Neola, and Neal D. Barnard, "Ketogenic diets and chronic disease: Weighing the benefits against the risks," *Frontiers in Nutrition* 8 (July 2021): 702802, doi: 10.3389/fnut.2021.702802.

This last comment was further underscored by my interview (October 4, 2022) with critical care professor Dr. Charles Sprung, who also identifies as an Orthodox Jew and has strictly practiced medicine according to Jewish Halacha (translated as "the way to behave"). He elaborated on Dr. Tulsky's position, stating, "The Jewish perspective is that nothing should be done to hasten the dying process—by a doctor or a patient. In my opinion and those of several of my colleagues [who are not Jewish], physicians should be curing and caring by providing palliative care but not . . . hastening death."

Dr. Sprung is Professor and Director Emeritus of the General ICU at Hadassah Hebrew University Medical Center in Jerusalem, and he was the chairman of the Medical and Scientific Subcommittee that contributed to the Israel Terminally Ill Law of 2005.[6] The law permits a competent, imminently dying person to refuse food and artificial feeding, and it requires the clinical staff to make a "reasonable effort" to persuade the person to eat and drink if he or she refuses.[7] According to Dr. Sprung, "If a person becomes incompetent, the law prohibits withholding food and fluid from the dying patient. Under these circumstances, doctors can provide food and fluids to a patient who had previously refused them."

He went on to say, "If, however, the doctor believes food or fluids would be harmful (e.g., by resulting in aspiration into the lungs) or the patient would suffer, then there is no obligation to provide the food and fluids."

But he then went on to say, "Regarding Dan, if he came to my attention, I would do everything in my power to prevent VSED and convince him of a better alternative."

Bioethicist Dr. Daniel Sulmasy would also dispute (email March 30, 2023) the morality of Dan employing VSED to die.[8] He has written that there are significant logical and ethical problems with the justifications generally offered for this practice,[9] and he points out that if there is no underlying pathological reason

---

[6] Rachel Nissanholtz-Gannot, Michal Gordon, and Ariel Yankellevich, "The Dying Patient Act: The letter of the law and implementation of the law," Myers Brookdale JDC, accessed October 4, 2022, https://brookdale-web.s3.amazonaws.com/uploads/2017/12/RR_734_17_English_summ ary.pdf.

[7] Charles L. Sprung, Margaret A. Somerville, Lukas Radbruch, et al., "Physician-assisted suicide and euthanasia: Emerging issues from a global perspective," J Palliative Care 33, no. 4 (October 2018): 197–203, doi: 10.1177/082585918777325.

[8] Daniel P. Sulmasy, "The ethics of medically assisted nutrition and hydration at the end of life: Separating the wheat from the chaff," in The Oxford Handbook of Ethics at the End of Life, eds. Stuart J. Youngner and Robert M. Arnold (New York: Oxford University Press, 2015), 126–153, doi: 10.1093/oxfordhb/9780199974412.013.14.

[9] Lynn A. Jansen and Daniel P. Sulmasy, "Sedation, alimentation, hydration, and equivocation: Careful conversation about care at the end of life," Annals of Internal Medicine 136, no. 11 (June 2002): 845–849, doi: 10.7326/0003-4819-136-11-200206040-00014.

why a person cannot eat (such as an inability to swallow), then "the act must be categorized as an act of killing." In his opinion, a truly respectful clinician ought not hesitate to challenge the patient's decision, "testing its depth, authenticity, and probity." To cooperate with a patient who follows this course of action is a form of "moral complicity," even when the practitioner is offering symptom control.

I reached out to Dr. Mark S. Komrad, MD, who has been a collaborator with Dr. Sprung, and who likewise argues against medical-assisted dying and euthanasia. But Dr. Komrad, who is a psychiatrist and medical ethicist on the faculty of Johns Hopkins University, the University of Maryland, and Tulane, also acknowledged that many physicians have different responses toward VSED. He wrote to me (October 7, 2022): "For those wishing to end their lives for whatever reason, VSED, is an ethical compromise which . . . does not involve asking a physician to violate an ethic that is venerable, critical, and deeply studied by medical professional groups. . . . VSED threads a needle in the contemporary conundrum between 'the right to die' of the patient and what it means to be a physician."

He continued, "A physician might legitimately tend the bedside of a patient pursuing VSED and provide comfort and the supportive continuity of the doctor–patient relationship in the face of the patient's choice and self-directed behavior. In VSED, the physician is indeed getting out of the way of death, not producing death. It might be emotionally uncomfortable and dissonant for some physicians, especially psychiatrists, to attend to a patient engaged in VSED. However, to be present at such a scenario would not be a violation of the values to which the doctor has 'professed' as a professional. Providing proximity, comfort and attendance, or what Dr. Paul Farmer calls 'accompaniment,' is a key virtue; the underlying message is 'I'll go with you and support you on your journey wherever it leads.' "[10]

*****

During a subsequent interview with John, I reviewed the recent events and started by asking, "So, if I'm up to date with things, then January 15 is no longer in the picture?

John said, "Correct."

"The decision to take a lethal overdose is gone, and instead you guys are actively pursuing VSED?"

[10] Susan Brink, "A million dollar prize for a doc who believes in 'accompaniment,'" NPR, December 16, 2020, https://www.npr.org/sections/goatsandsoda/2020/12/16/946740727/dr-paul-farmer-was-surprised-to-get-a-million-dollar-philosophy-prize.

"Correct, again."

"Do you have reason to think that VSED will be any more tolerable to the people who objected to the original plan?"

"No. We don't know how they're going to respond, but this is the option that the family left us. There is nothing legal that anyone can do to prevent Dan from going ahead with this."

"Okay," I said. "But the intent now is to *not* make this announcement to the family until things have further developed and the details of the new plan are clearer?"

"Yes," he said.

But Dan couldn't help himself from communicating with his loved ones. Fortunately, a couple of days later, John reported that the Winter family dynamics had begun to shift. As word spread that Dan was now considering VSED rather than an overdose, a greater sense of calm was returning to the extended clan—at least from John and Dan's perspectives.

The couple had begun discussing when to initiate the fast, and they spent a couple of hours on the phone with the hospice coordinator from the insurance company. She assured them that Dan would be accepted to her program *after* he became symptomatic. However, the otherwise physically fit man was less than ecstatic when she reported that one of their patients survived for 4 weeks before dying. Dan was eager to begin what he called, "the countdown." He hoped that it would take at most 7 days before he became drowsy enough to have to remain in bed.

Multiple articles in the medical literature,[11,12,13,14] as well as position statements issued by national and international professional healthcare societies

[11] Timothy Quill, Linda Ganzini, Robert D. Truog, and Thaddeus Mason Pope, "Voluntarily stopping eating and drinking among patients with serious advanced illness: Clinical, ethical, and legal aspects," *JAMA Internal Medicine* 178, no. 1 (January 2018): 123–127, doi:10.1001/jamainternmed.2017.6307.

[12] T. E. Quill, B. Lo, and D. W. Brock, "Palliative options of last resort: A comparison of voluntarily stopping eating and drinking, terminal sedation, physician-assisted suicide, and voluntary active euthanasia," *JAMA* 278, no. 23 (December 1997): 2099–2104, doi: 10.1001/jama.278.23.2099.

[13] Eva E. Bolt, Martijn Hagens, Dick Willems, and Bregje D. Onwuteaka-Philipsen, "Primary care patients hastening death by voluntarily stopping eating and drinking," *Annals of Family Medicine* 13, no. 5 (September 2015): 421–428, doi: 10.1370/afm.1814.

[14] Takuya Shinjo, Tatsuya Morita, Daisuke Kiuchi, et al., "Japanese physicians' experiences of terminally ill patients voluntarily stopping eating and drinking: A national survey," *BMJ Supportive & Palliative Care* 9, no. 2 (June 2019): 143–145, doi: 10.1136/bmjspcare-2017-001426.

have been published on the subject of VSED.[15,16] Recently, a clinical guideline was completed in the United States,[17] along with the forementioned first comprehensive textbook.[18] The latter is thoughtful and balanced, and its editors have written: "In sum, VSED provides an opportunity to achieve a relatively peaceful, personally controlled death for patients seeking an escape from the prospect of unacceptable suffering or deterioration in their present condition or foreseeable future."

I couldn't help being struck by the phrase, "Relatively peaceful." *Relative peaceful?* I asked myself.

[15] Lukas Radbruch and Liliana De Lima, "International Association for Hospice and Palliative Care response regarding voluntary cessation of food and water," *Journal of Palliative Medicine* 20, no. 6 (June 2017): 578–579, doi: 10.1089/jpm.2017.0077, Epub 2017 Mar 28, PMID: 28350515.

[16] T. E. Quill and I. R. Byock, "Responding to intractable terminal suffering: The role of terminal sedation and voluntary refusal of food and fluids. ACP-ASIM End-of-Life Care Consensus Panel," *Annals of Internal Medicine* 132, no. 5 (March 2000): 408–414, doi: 10.7326/0003-4819-132-5-200003070-00012.

[17] H. Wechkin, R. Macauley, P. T. Menzel, P. L. Reagan, N. Simmers, and T. E. Quill. "Clinical guidelines for voluntarily stopping eating and drinking (VSED)," *Journal of Pain and Symptom Management* 2023, https://doi.org/10.1016/j.jpainsymman.2023.06.016.

[18] Timothy E. Quill, Paul T. Menzel, Thaddeus M. Pope, and Judith K. Schwarz, "Best practices, enduring challenges, and opportunities for VSED," in *Voluntarily Stopping Eating and Drinking: A Compassionate, Widely Available Option for Hastening Death*, eds. Timothy E. Quill, Paul T. Menzel, Thaddeus M. Pope, and Judith K. Schwarz (New York: Oxford University Press, 2021), 129.

24

Numerous phone calls with nephews, nieces, and other family members ensued, and a relieved Dan reported, "I have stopped thinking that I am heading up Mt. Calvary with a cross on my back." He was now confident the family would support his choice, and Dan felt reassured that hospice personnel were familiar with voluntarily stopping eating and drinking (VSED) and prepared to help. The hospice coordinator clarified that her staff would step in at the point when he was no longer walking or talking. "I'm sure they want to be confident it's a real thing—an actual fast with no cheating," Dan said. He arranged for an appointment with his primary care physician to obtain medications to alleviate any discomfort that might occur before hospice took over. Dan was ready to begin VSED.

I asked, "Are you going to announce the date?"

"I'm not going to do that again," he said. "It was ill-advised. . . . I'm telling people it's probably next week sometime, and I'm letting that percolate through. . . . My family is large and raucous and good and bad and ugly and pretty . . . and I've always felt loved."

However, his voice dropped an octave as he said, "I'm trying not to be bitter about it, but I was so disappointed by the reaction of some of these folks. I don't want to say, 'lack of respect' . . . but my decision hit them in a way I didn't anticipate, and they must have felt blindsided."

Several family members who upset him apologized and expressed remorse. However, a few others informed Dan that they unequivocally would *not* speak with him while he continued to pursue *any* plan to foreshorten his life, including VSED. I wasn't sure whether Dan was being ironic or earnest when he said, "This is not a good time for me to hold grudges."

Dan was pleased to keep the timing just a little vague, in part because he didn't want anyone to arrive for a final visit during COVID. He told a few friends that if he allowed someone to come to the condominium, "there's no way you can avoid hugging people on their deathbed . . . and I'd be so nervous about spreading the infection that I wouldn't be able to have a peaceful death."

Dan was also glad he had been approached by his brother-in-law, Steven Stingley, who began interviewing him on the phone with the goal of writing Dan's story for the family. "Here's a microphone," Steven told him, "and you get to talk to me—somebody who loves you, has known you since we were in high school, and who is married to your sister. I'm going to ask you all these questions, and you get to say whatever you want."

"We've been talking," Dan said, "and there have been moments of catharsis. My sisters are in the peanut gallery, listening in. We've had a lot of fun. It's like the golden ticket to narcissism land."

One of Dan's obsessions remained the social and political ramifications of the new method he was now planning on using to die. He said, "VSED is interesting, and this is an opportunity for people to learn about it. There are members of the family who would cringe if it said 'suicide' on my death certificate, as opposed to VSED or dementia." He only half-humorously observed to me that the words "complications of Alzheimer's" might be the most acceptable.

Dan was unaware that some hospices are becoming more willing to receive patients for VSED,[1] and they may rely on a terminal diagnosis of "dehydration" and then list the cause on death certificates as being "secondary to cessation of caloric and food intake, and secondary to . . . Alzheimer's, ALS, or Parkinson's, etc." Some members of the medical and hospice community find VSED more acceptable than physician-assisted dying because the method itself relieves concerns that a person is acting impulsively or under coercion.[2] Anyone who is resolute enough to persist in VSED has demonstrated that they are exceedingly determined.

*****

"Dan," I said, "You changed your plan. I'm curious whether you *still* think that for people who are dealing with Alzheimer's the idea of shortening life by taking an overdose that is *not* medically supervised is something which should be considered an option?"

He replied, "Oh, definitely. I changed methods for several distinct reasons, but that doesn't mean that I wouldn't support somebody taking their life in another manner."

He continued, "I want to promote the idea it's okay to feel like you don't want to live with this disease. It's really okay. There are a lot of us out there.

[1] Jim Rough, "Jean had both Alzheimer's disease and Lewy body dementia . . . And a GOOD DEATH," Final Exit Network, accessed October 16, 2022, https://www.thegooddeathsocietyblog. net/2022/10/16/jean-had-both-alzheimers-disease-and-lewy-body-dementia-and-a-good-death/.

[2] Susan Stefan, *Rational Suicide, Irrational Law: Examining Current Approaches to Suicide in Policy and Law* (New York: Oxford University Press, 2016).

There are nonpainful and nonviolent options. Pharmaceuticals are one of them. It is not my intention to be the least bit hesitant about ending your life with pharmaceuticals."

Bioethicists have long debated the permissibility of suicide for those facing dementia's malevolent effects.[3,4,5,6] Some philosophers have argued that rational suicide is nothing short of selfishness run amok, myopic individualism, an unrealistic belief in autonomy, and an assault on the normal bonds of family and community. Others have gone so far as to conclude that, in accordance with a Kantian interpretation, people who develop dementias have a *moral obligation* to kill themselves. This last hypothesis is the sort that leads nonphilosophers, like me, to wonder whether those bioethicists are accompanying Alice in Wonderland.[7,8]

And then there is Dena S. Davis, JD, PhD, Professor Emerita at Cleveland-Marshall College of Law and the Endowed Presidential Chair in Health, Humanities, and Social Sciences at Lehigh University, who argues that it is morally defensible—not obligatory—to end one's life in the face of impending incompetence. She has written in support of *preemptive suicide* in the context of Alzheimer's disease[9] and begins by questioning why people fear the illness and how individuals who express interest in rational suicide usually do so from a mixture of motivations that are related to autonomy (e.g., distaste for a life of dependence), nonmaleficence (e.g., a wish to avoid burdening others), and beneficence (e.g., the preservation of assets to pass along).

When we spoke (December 22, 2022, interview), she confided that this position was forged by the experience with her own mother, "one of the fiercest, most autonomy-focused persons you will ever meet." But Professor Davis's mother *denied she had Alzheimer's from the day she was diagnosed to her eventual death some 10 years later.* (Dr. Kluger would have cited this as a perfect example

---

[3] Dennis R. Cooley, "Response to open peer commentaries on 'A Kantian moral duty for the soon to be demented to commit suicide,'" *American Journal of Bioethics* 7, no. 6 (2007): 1–3, doi: 10.1080/15265160701429607.

[4] Katerina Standish, *Why Not Suicide? Suicide Through a Peacebuilding Lens* (New York: Springer, 2020), 213–239, doi:10.1007/978-981-13-9737-0_8.

[5] Alan Jotkowitz, "Is there life not worthy of living?," *American Journal of Bioethics* 7, no. 6 (June 2007): 62–63, doi: 10.1080/15265160701347569.

[6] Brian M. Draper, "Suicidal behavior and assisted suicide in dementia," *International Psychogeriatrics* 27, no. 10 (October 2015): 1601–1611, doi:10.1017/S1041610215000629.

[7] Dennis R. Cooley, "A Kantian moral duty for the soon-to-be demented to commit suicide," *American Journal of Bioethics* 7, no. 6 (June 2007): 37–44, doi: 10.1080/15265160701347478.

[8] John Hardwig, "Is there a duty to die?," *Hastings Center Reports* 27, no. 2 (March-April 1997): 34–42, PMID: 9131351.

[9] Dena S. Davis, "Alzheimer disease and pre-emptive suicide," *Journal of Medical Ethics* 40, no. 8 (August 2014): 543–549, doi: 10.1136/medethics-2012-101022.

of anosognosia.) During that decade, there were numerous exit ramps—*natural* and *unnatural*—that Professor Davis could have used to grant her mother the kind of death the woman had always previously evinced wanting. However, she told me, "I couldn't take them. I doubt anybody really could."

I never discussed Professor Davis's view with Dan, but he was of the opinion that people should be accorded access to the necessary information for arranging quick and painless rational suicides. "I think people ought to be able to have the opportunity," he told me. "It may make me seem like an unbalanced radical, and I've been accused of that before," he chortled, "but I feel very strongly about this."

Dan believed that it makes no sense "to bankrupt our society . . . people with dementias are dying long and awful deaths . . . with no humanity left. . . . I wish there was a way to say the word, *suicide*, and describe somebody like me. I wish that word wasn't so fraught."

Unknown to Dan, John, and me, a nationwide poll was taking place while we were having this conversation. Sponsored by the Final Exit Network (FEN), over a thousand people were surveyed to explore how Americans feel about hastening death rather than enduring the full consequences of dementia.[10] Forty-four percent of respondents endorsed a position that competent individuals diagnosed with early-stage dementia should have access to a peaceful method to end life before losing capacity, 31% were neutral or unsure about the idea, and 24% opposed it. Just over half of respondents, 53%, supported the idea that *competent* individuals with early-stage dementia should be able to legally stipulate, for their future *incompetent* selves, that they wanted food and drink withdrawn and for doctors to participate in keeping them comfortable. Only 15% opposed this practice.

The poll data suggest that when it comes to accelerating death in the context of dementia, supporters currently outnumber opponents, but there is a fair number of people who are uncertain. "This subject's coming up more and more," Dan said. "It's gaining momentum, and I'm thrilled."

*****

Dan shifted to talking about medical assistance in dying (MAiD) and how, in the United States and several other countries, people with dementia face a Catch-22: in the earlier stages of the disease, they have the mental capacity to request voluntary assisted dying but do not meet strict eligibility criteria because their death is not imminent. But as the dementia progresses, they are shut out of the protocols because of their inability to meaningfully consent.

---

[10] "Americans want option to hasten death if faced with dementia," Final Exit Network, accessed October 3, 2022, https://finalexitnetwork.org/news-events/dementia-poll/.

He reiterated his hope that it will only be a matter of time before America's aid-in-dying laws are revised to empower and include this sector of the population. The neglect had gone on too long. Which is why I was delighted to later encounter (May 16, 2023, interview) Janet Hager, the secretary of a newly formed Californian nonprofit group called A Better Exit.

While grateful that the state has legalized physician-assisted dying, the organization members believe that the law is overly restrictive. They are convinced it is time to shift from the 26-year-old Oregon template to a new set of criteria that will be more inclusive of people with neurodegenerative disorders.

A Better Exit is trying to alter California's current statute in three ways: (1) by broadening MAiD eligibility criteria to include individuals suffering from grievous and irremediable diseases and have a life expectancy greater than 6 months, (2) allowing persons the choice to self-ingest or receive an intravenous infusion when using MAiD, and (3) letting people with early to mid-stage dementia be evaluated for and have access to MAiD when two physicians determine they retain capacity.

"Why," I inquired of Hager, "did you arrive at those specific changes to the law?"

"Well, eliminating the 6-month criteria made sense because it feels like it's an arbitrary number. Plus, Lew, you are a physician, so you also know that sometimes it's really hard to prognosticate with any kind of accuracy.

"Second, we'd like to see an option of having something injectable, because many people with disorders, such as advanced Parkinson's, multiple sclerosis, and ALS [amyotrophic lateral sclerosis], may not be able to swallow or push a plunger. So, we feel that there should be an intravenous option.

"Lastly, people like Dan, with early to mid-stage dementias, often have capacity and should at least be evaluated and assessed for medical aid in dying. If they've maintained capacity, then they shouldn't be excluded."

25

On January 16, I spoke with John. It was his 70th birthday. "Sometimes," I said, "it just seems sardonic and even cruel to say something like, 'Happy Birthday!'"

"I know, I know," said John. "But each of them is a biggie, especially because, in 1989, the first HIV doc I saw told me, 'You need to get your papers in order now. You need to do whatever traveling you want to do now, because you're going to die soon.'"

"So, 32 years later, at age 70, what have you learned?" I asked.

"I have come to appreciate the limits of medical knowledge."

I chuckled ruefully.

"I've learned how to ask for help," he said, "and I have learned that there are different kinds of love. I've had the good fortune of experiencing many of them—and not just the romantic versions. I have learned how to build my logical family." He paused for a moment and then inquired, "Do you know the distinction between a biological family and a logical family?"

"I do not."

"It's a phrase that was developed by Armistead Maupin, the San Francisco writer, who recounted the fictional story of a group of people who lived in San Francisco leading up to and during the AIDS epidemic. There was a character who owned a boarding house, and she was very careful about who she selected to live there because they became her 'logical family.' After having experienced rejection to one degree or another from their biological families, they were transformed by becoming part of each other's logical family."

"Oh."

"I, too, piece-by-piece-by-piece, put together a family that has sustained me ever since I came out. It began as a group of gay men, then a lesbian couple, and now a number of straight people—several of whom were originally my architecture-design clients. More recently, they include various members of the arts community. There are only a few of the original gay men who have survived, and while we're not necessarily as close as we were, they are the people who I can call upon at any point. We stay in touch. Their understanding of what we have all endured is entirely different from that of anybody who merely observed it."

John recognized that the epidemic profoundly molded him, but equally important was his relative isolation during the first 28 years of his life—a reaction to the awareness of being homosexual. He explained, "I was so afraid to reveal myself to people. But once I began to do that and found people who loved me and people who I loved back . . . well, I got pretty good at opening up. . . ."

Once again, I felt moved by John's confidence in me. I appreciated that he was entrusting me with his story, as well as that of Dan's. John had been through a type of purgatory that I could barely imagine. As a psychiatrist, I have met with enough people suffering from deep and abiding depressions to know—at least as an observer—how monstrous life can feel under such circumstances. Although I had witnessed the AIDS epidemic, it was only indirectly. From his more immediate and intimate perspective, John watched how friends and lovers were disfigured and savaged by an unfeeling virus. I admired him for having created his extensive logical family and for the special qualities that made him such an attractive human being.

"I think that Dan is lucky to have you as a husband and friend," I said.

Abruptly changing topics, John then told me that one of the unexpected benefits of deciding to switch to voluntarily stopping eating and drinking (VSED) came in the form of a phone call he had with his own sister, a retired hospice nurse, who said, "I'm on your team. I can fully support you and Dan."

"Dan and I then had a long conversation with my sister," John said, "and she can be quite blunt and gentle at the same time. Having worked in this field for a long time, she's developed really good interpersonal skills and has plenty of practical expertise. Dan got to hear from her what the entire VSED process might look like. She also encouraged me to promptly begin establishing my own care team. The first friends I contacted are a couple of men who live six blocks away from us, and they immediately said, 'We'll give you a key to our condo, and cocktails start at 6:30 every night, and dinner is promptly served at 7:00.' I have since spoken to four other friends who have each spontaneously offered to provide anything I need."

John was buoyed up at the thought of tapping his logical family for supportive companionship during the upcoming ordeal. In addition, he recognized the necessity of finding someone who was willing to spend a few hours a day with Dan so that he could take a break and step away from the condo. He was disinclined to ask any of his "second or third circle of friends"—most of whom were close to his age, "Because, the last thing I want to do is put them in a position of saying, 'Yup, I will help you,' when what they are really thinking is, *Sorry, but I'm afraid of COVID*."

I then asked John about the dissension that gripped the Winter clan, and he said, "Most people in our society have *not* reflected on life and death, and they work as hard as they can to *not* do so. I've had to pull myself up to the 5,000-foot level and look at this as a three-dimensional puzzle." He went on to say, "I know that Dan and I can only influence the people around us so much."

John paused for a moment to collect his thoughts and then said, "You asked me what have I learned on this birthday? Well, it is preferable to look at things straight on, rather than approaching stuff obliquely. For better or for worse that's what we're doing—tackling this as directly as we can."

*****

On Thursday, January 21, I connected again with Dan, who began the interview by saying, "Hi, Lew. I was talking to my 88-year-old mother, and she had a stroke few days ago. Mom won't be able to walk. She won't be able to get out of bed. It's kind of the last lap."

"Literally," I quipped, and immediately regretted my feeble attempt at gallows humor. I embarrassedly muttered, "Oh, man!"

Dan chose to ignore my reaction, and he said, "It's too bad, but she's had a long life and is ready to go."

"What did she say on the phone?"

"Oh, we were talking about anything . . . nonsense . . . about eating in bed, and how her other caregiver comes in when she needs to shower and bathe. Mom's taking it all pretty well. She sounds like a drunk, but she's laughing about it. It involves her left side. She was lying on her back and couldn't lift her left arm to touch her chin."

Dan went on. "We're making a decision each day whether or not to tell her what's happening with me. My sister and my cousin and my ex-wife are concocting a plan. The current thinking is, after I die, she'll be told, 'Dan fell into a coma.' However, my preference is to let her know the truth immediately when I decide upon the date to begin fasting. If I was her, I would want to know. I'd be a little disappointed if my kids didn't think I could handle it. But it's not my responsibility, and everybody else is going to have to live with it. I've got way too much going on right now."

He resumed, "My mother's pretty great. If you met her, she would immediately ask, 'Are you married?' 'How many children do you have?' 'What do you do for a living?' 'Did you graduate college?' 'Where do you shop?' 'What's your favorite kind of food?' Then she'd ask you over for dinner, and you'd be in the dining room that same night."

"Are you really different from her? I'd guess that pretty much describes you, too, doesn't it?" I inquired.

"Yeah," he said. "But I wouldn't ask about your education level. I'd be a little bit more discreet."

Dan's thinking then got noticeably more scattered, and when I remarked about my difficulty following his train of thought, he said, "I had another episode last week in which I couldn't recognize where I was." Once again it took place while he was walking his dog around the park, and this time he relied on the ever-faithful Friday to lead the way back home.

"Also, I'm dropping a lot of things," he said. "I was eating and dropped a hamburger yesterday. I don't know why this is happening, except that it's part of the disease." He was clearly embarrassed and didn't appear to fully appreciate that Alzheimer's frequently robs its victims of their motor skills. No further explanation was really necessary.

And then with no preamble, Dan said, "VSED is beginning tomorrow."

I wasn't entirely surprised by his declaration as much as pleased that he had imparted the decision to me.

Dan said: "I worry a little bit about whether I'm going to be able to do this. I want to utilize every pain reliever and antianxiety medication that I can. I've gotten 11 tabs of Ativan (a minor tranquilizer). I don't know if that's going to be enough. My primary physician has been balking at getting me a referral to hospice." Dan couldn't understand his doctor's hesitance, but he had sought and found someone else to make the official referral.

I asked, "As you approach the first day of not eating and drinking, where are you at?"

"I'm resolved," he emphatically said. "I'm relieved that John and I have hired our personal trainer to help. We are very fond of Sean. Because 24-hour coverage is needed, we've got hospice for a few hours, John will take some hours, and Sean will have his own schedule. We have had a really great response from friends. The neighbors are cleaning out a couple of shelves of their refrigerators, so John can put his food in there and come over and eat. He's got keys to the condos of two different couples who each want him to freely come and go. One of the couples has dinner at 6:30 and drinks at 7:00," Dan told me, slightly mixing up the details, which he was intermittently doing throughout this interview. "They are going to cook for him every night," Dan said, "regardless of whether he's coming over."

"Good. You have made plans both for John's support along with your own?"

"Yeah. The way I look at it, this first phase involves less care for me and more care for him. I'll need some attention to stay focused. I'm quite confident that it's going to work. I don't know how uncomfortable it's going to be. I'm hoping not too much."

I asked, "Do you have a clearer idea now about the hospice and when they will actually begin coming to offer their services?"

"The hospice intake nurse spent a chunk of time with me on the phone," he said with evident enthusiasm. "She kept repeating, 'We're going to do *everything you need*.' She made us feel confident that they knew what they were doing and had oodles of experience."

"My understanding," I said, "was that the hospice intended to wait until you became more symptomatic, and they would then expect a call from you or John to initiate things?"

"Yes," he said. "That's the Medicare protocol they will be following. Even though I'm not a Medicare patient, they're obligated to follow Medicare guidelines for the initiation of hospice. They need to have a 6-month or less prognosis, and after I can't walk and talk that'll satisfy the requirements."

Dan and I arranged for the next interview. He understood that I was scheduled to speak with John in a couple of days, and we agreed to reconnect 2 days after that interview. I admittedly felt ambivalent about calling him when VSED had begun, not wanting to take up his time while he was in the process of actively dying. But he said, "Don't hesitate to try to reach me, because I'll be at home and wanting to talk."

I repeated his words, "You'll be home and wanting to talk."

"You bet," he said.

"I will call. Meantime, I will speak with John on Saturday."

"Alright. Perfect. Thank you!"

"Hey, Dan," I said. "Take care."

"Bye, Lew."

"Bye-bye."

I didn't know it, but those would be our last words.

26

When next I spoke with John, he explained that Dan had lovingly prepared their final meal of sweet and sour chicken before beginning the fast. The leftovers were carefully wrapped and placed in the freezer.

On the first day of voluntarily stopping eating and drinking (VSED), other than a caffeine-withdrawal headache, things went smoothly. Dan spent a fair amount of time on the phone speaking with friends and family. Several of the Winter women assumed primary responsibility for dealing with his mother, and they helped disseminate updates to the clan.

"Our friend, Sean," John said, "came over yesterday to learn where he's going to park and how to use the fob to get into the building. He hung out with Dan while I left and did some errands. All of that went well. Our next-door neighbors here in the condo invited me to eat with them every night. I accepted their offer and had dinner the first night out on the terrace, which was beautiful. The food was delicious, and the conversation was both serious and distracting. It was really great.

"The difficulties we had at the beginning of this process with family members," he explained, "are beginning to fade because Dan is getting touching expressions of support for what he's doing."

I would learn later that the situation was not so straightforward when I spoke with Wynne, Dan's ex-wife, who said: "I realized that I was *not* going to be able to change his mind. . . . If he went through with it, I wanted him to know that I loved him and supported him. I did *not* support his decision but supported his right to decide."

"John," I asked, "when you went to the neighbors and had dinner with them, was this because you didn't want to cook and produce food odors in your apartment that might bother Dan?"

"Yup." John paused and cleared his throat, and then said, "that was the impetus. I had read this advice on various websites about VSED. We're not going to do the most extreme version, but the refrigerator is presently empty of anything edible, and I have begun drinking a cold-brew coffee with no fragrance."

The social activist and bioethicist Sarah Kiskadden-Bechtel found it poignant to realize that smells, an otherwise normal part of everyday life, had become something that the two men were deftly trying to side-step and control (email, March 14, 2023).

"Dan is now using sugar-free lozenges for dry mouth, along with Biotene mouthwash and spray," John went on. "We have mouth swabs, and I've continued to be in touch with the hospice by phone. I feel confident there's always someone in reach. The hospice staff are available, and they appear to be professional, caring, and compassionate."

Although Dan had desired "a quick, quiet, calm ending . . . through pharmaceuticals," the two men had come to understand that the word "suicide" was "a big neon sign with deeply negative, religiously based, cultural connotations."

John hoped someone might coin a more neutral or positive phrase to capture the desire of people, like Dan, to take control over the end of life. "Self-deliverance" is a term that works for some folk, but I, and many others of my generation, associate *deliverance* with either religion or the 1972 survival-thriller movie starring Jon Voight in the Georgia backcountry—the one with the "Dueling Banjos" soundtrack. Not exactly ideal connotations.

After beginning the fast, Dan continued taking Friday out for his walks. These were meaningful, twice-daily rituals. But Dan had begun to feel increasingly weary, and he realized that the dog walks soon would soon become impossible. He had started taking naps lasting up to 3 ½ hours. Otherwise, from John's perspective, Dan had not developed any serious complications or side effects.

"There just isn't a polite protocol to address Dan's condition and VSED," John said. "When I have told our closest friends, everybody expresses shock that the fasting has started—mainly because due to the pandemic they hadn't seen him since March of last year. . . . Once they understand what the dementia symptoms have become—and primarily the one involving walking the dog three blocks away and not having any idea where he is—they can understand. That became the marker for Dan. He doesn't really want to know what the next symptom will be. He does not want to further lose his autonomy."

John said, "Most of our friends have grasped what's happening. They say to me, 'Tell Dan that I love him and fully support what he's doing, and I wish there were more things I could provide.' 'I wish I could come and hold you both,' is a regular refrain. Our friends aren't disappointed with his decision, and they want Dan to know the huge impact that he's had on their lives."

*****

When I called Dan's cell for our next scheduled appointment, it was John who answered. Dan had relinquished the phone.

"Dan is not really up to having a conversation," he said, "so I wanted to update you. Yesterday, was day 4 and he slept for 12 ½ hours. Arrangements had been made for him to telephone his mother in Kansas City. His ex-wife, Wynne, and several others were to be on the call and by her bedside." Dan insisted that his mother be told the complete truth, and, after the call finished, he told John, "So that's what we did. We let her know the truth."

John remarked, "He was very happy that the truth became the chosen option."

I said, "It is consistent with who your husband is."

"Correct," said John, "and it is reassuring that after all that's happened, these family members respected his wish. Their respect is very important to both of us."

On the following day, both men took Friday for a last walk together. But it required more energy and concentration than Dan could continue to muster, and John left him afterward in bed with the dog in attendance. Dan was clearly more infirm, and his speech was becoming less directed, less comprehensible. Earlier in the week, multiple emails, texts, letters, cards, and bouquets arrived at the apartment. Dan tried to respond but this had become impossible.

Hunger was not an issue, and he dealt with thirst by sucking on the lozenges, swishing mouthwash, and using moist swabs. He was still independently moving around, but much more slowly and carefully.

John had just broadcast the news that in all likelihood Dan would not be able to speak with family members again. Another half a day without food and water, and John doubted his capacity to respond appropriately.

"If people call," John said, "I can certainly put the phone up to his ear and let as many of them say, 'I love you,' as will want to."

I said, "I can hear in your voice, John, the anguish you're going through as these things are progressing. You are having to play a more active role and make decisions that otherwise Dan would have been the one to make."

He replied, "It's really so counter to everything we've ever been to each other. I have never had to speak for Dan before. He has continued to acknowledge, as recently as last night before we went to bed and before I left to have dinner with the neighbors, that he knows how hard this is for me. He is so grateful. He said, 'I just don't know if I could have done this without you.' I know he means it. Then he rolled over and instantly fell asleep."

*****

I spoke again with John the following day, and he was thrilled to have received a call from Dan's mother.

"We had this lovely, lovely conversation," John said. "She wanted me to know how much it meant to her and the family that I am here for Dan."

"How much it meant to her? Oh, that is amazing."

"She recognizes that it is not easy, and she called to console me."

"Wow! This from a mother who is losing her son."

"Yes, and her voice was strong and clear. She said, 'Okay now, I want to make sure you're really listening to what I'm going to say next. Are you listening?' So, I replied, 'Yes.' And she said, 'You are a gift to Dan. You are a gift to this family.' And then, 'Please call me. Please stay in touch.' It was just great."

I said, "It sounds like Dan was correct in pushing Wynne, and his sister, and the others to level with her and tell the truth."

"The minute I met Dan's mother," John said, "she literally and metaphorically embraced me. She said, 'We're your family now.' She has never treated me any differently. So that's not out of character for her. She's always been a very lively, engaging person. I think she speaks as easily to people who work at the post office as she would to the governor."

"I certainly felt our conversation today went well," he continued. "I was sobbing but responded as best I could. She really wasn't interested in my telling her too much. Dan had talked to her yesterday afternoon. They're speaking with each other with this clear understanding of what's going on. So, it's just about as good as it can possibly be."

John and I reviewed how the other family members were responding. Several had entirely severed their connection and wanted no further communication with Dan unless he changed the position about ending his life. We both found this stance to be tragic.

After speaking together for an hour, I said, "Listen. This may be the right moment for us to stop today. I just looked out the window, and it appears as if we've just had three inches of beautiful, fluffy, snow. I'm pretty excited about this storm." I also knew that in a short while there would be a waxing gibbous moon suspended over my neighborhood.

"Oh, lucky you," John said.

"So, I'm going to take a walk and think about what we've talked about. Perhaps we can continue on an every-other-day schedule for now. If at our next call, Dan is up to saying, 'Howdy,' would you put him on the phone?"

"Yup."

"I appreciate being kept apprised about what's going on. I loved hearing about the conversation you had with Dan's mother."

"She was sweet. . . . Lew, speak to you again soon."

27

John reported that on day 8 of the fast, Dan tried to stay awake and remain alert during a visit from the hospice's nurse, a muscular, heavily tattooed, soft-spoken, young man. Since Dan started voluntarily stopping eating and drinking (VSED), John had been regularly checking in with the hospice, and his description of Dan's latest symptoms prompted the nurse's evaluation. Unfortunately, the man with the brightly colored tats decided to *not* officially initiate hospice services— because the patient appeared to still be too perky. It was clear, however, that Dan would soon qualify.

On day 9 of his fast, Dan became disoriented and incoherent, and hospice services were begun. A couple of hours later, a hospital bed and a walker were delivered to the apartment. Shortly afterward, additional antianxiety medications and some morphine arrived, along with instructions for their administration.

John explained to me that Dan never ended up using the hospital bed or the walker. Had he lingered longer, the bed would have been necessary to be able to turn him more easily and prevent bed sores. Hospice did not provide any staff, other than the nurse, who telephoned a couple of times to check up on Dan's condition. The nurse made VSED seem normal, he was consistently encouraging, and the arrival of an assortment of additional medications was greatly appreciated.

Friday, the labradoodle, didn't leave Dan's side except to go out for walks or to gobble down a meal. She was sweetly attentive, placing her face right up against his and maintaining eye contact for up to 15 minutes at a time. It was a staring contest that Dan would usually lose by falling asleep.

Dan was unable to meaningfully participate in phone calls, and John assumed total responsibility for keeping the family up to date about his condition. Either Sean or another friend briefly spelled John, who would mainly take those opportunities to pop out for some lunch or dinner.

"Well, this has been such a different process than we originally anticipated," John told me. "I guess it has its own benefits, in that his sweetness, the essence of who he is, remains present. When I tell him I love him, his eyes brighten a little bit. He can say, 'I love you, too,' but he's just . . . there's just less of him all the time. I don't know if that's easier or not. It's just what it is at this point."

John summed up the situation: "His conviction remains strong. He's completely determined, but he's also ready for this to be over. . . . I just don't know how his bodily systems are able to continue functioning."

Dan was producing minimal urine and not moving his bowels. He seemed to want to sleep as much as possible and was taking a small dose of a tranquilizer every few hours.

*****

Dan's situation stands in contrast to a *New England Journal of Medicine* piece entitled, "Learning about end-of-life care from Grandpa."[1] A palliative medicine physician, Scott D. Halpern, wrote: "For people with a consistent desire to end their life . . . [stopping] eating and drinking is just too challenging. Hospice experts around the country had warned me that less than 20 percent of people who try to do so 'succeed,' with most reversing course because of vicious thirst."

Other doctors, like Jerald Sanders (interview on October 15, 2022), the medical director of Whidbey Health Hospice Care in Washington State, dispute this figure—although, admittedly, his experience with VSED is based on only having seen a handful of patients. He explained to me: "Locally, our hospices will admit someone on day 5 of VSED either with a specific medical diagnosis (if available) or malnutrition. Dealing with the anxieties, beliefs, prejudices of friends and family members around the entire subject of VSED is never ending. I sincerely believe hospice care is appropriate and that symptoms can be managed, usually with minimal medication."

Palliative care clinicians and others who care for the dying appreciate that most of their time and effort needs to be expended on issues that standardized protocols can't address. Much, if not most, of their attention often needs to be focused on educating and stabilizing the family caregivers and individual loved ones.

On day 10, I asked John, "To be concrete about this, did you ever hear Dan say, 'I'm thirsty. Maybe I'll take a drink?'"

"I heard him say he was thirsty, but he entered into the process knowing that he was going to be thirsty."

I persisted and asked, "But he never once said, 'So, get me a glass of water or orange juice?'"

[1] Scott D. Halpern, "Learning about end-of-life care from Grandpa," *New England Journal of Medicine* 384, no. 5 (February 2021): 400–401, doi: 10.1056/NEJMp2026629.

"Correct. Oddly, back when Dan was going to take the pharmaceutical over-dose, he had been looking forward to having a glass of vodka or a vodka tonic as part of the lethal cocktail. One night, Dan again mentioned missing that final drink. So, we made a vodka tonic with a slice of lemon. Dan then took one sip, luxuriated in the experience, carefully spat out the mouthful, and put the glass aside. A single sip was all he needed. He was completely committed to VSED, not relapsing on alcohol, and not prolonging his life whatsoever."

At this point in his fast, Dan was having constant headaches, and the hospice staff considered administering morphine.

"He is restless, and as a result I haven't slept well for a couple of nights," John told me. "I feel a little bit numb, although there are lots of different emotions right beneath the surface."

"Yes?"

"I'm not interested in chatting with friends and family. I've been doing minimal texting twice a day to let his sister and ex-wife know what's going on. A couple of friends have texted me, and I try to return all of those."

"And Dan?"

"He's ready. His desire to communicate is pretty much gone. He doesn't want to chat, nor do I try to make him."

"What is that like, the fact that he can't even speak with you?"

"I feel terribly helpless. I wish I could make all his pain and discomfort go away, but I haven't been able to do that with what we have at our disposal. It's my great hope that hospice is bringing more medications."

I asked John, "What else are you going through emotionally?"

He answered, "I have to admit that I am feeling a little angry about what the nurse had said a few days ago—that Dan didn't qualify to start hospice."

"Explain this a bit more?" I asked.

"None of these hospice rules were written to cover precisely what Dan is going through. They really are based on people dying from cancer or whatever diseases typically end people's lives. So, there's kind of a sense that because Dan brought this on himself there's no need to lessen his suffering."

John continued, "That's my emotional response to what's going on. It's not my intellectual response. I understand that there are rules and reasons."

"Tell me if I'm getting this correct," I said, "are you saying that the symptom management protocols and the initiation of hospice have been established for certain situations, like end-stage carcinomas? However, it is high time this was changed and expanded to reflect the situations of people, like Dan, who have dementias and want to employ VSED?"

"Yup," John replied. "No question about it. Because VSED is still relatively uncommon, we haven't set up a solid system to anticipate its symptoms and palliate them."

John continued, "But there's more. I hope there will be people who read this story and say it's well past the time for accommodating people with dementing illnesses and making VSED seem like a primitive alternative."

"A primitive alternative?"

"For people with dementia being able to take control over the end of their lives. It's time from my perspective that we create a path for folk in the early stages of dementia which will offer them easier access to a pharmaceutical end— a simple and painless overdose."

"Go on," I said to John.

"I understand there will need to be a protocol, perhaps not unlike what people go through now to qualify for the Oregon Death with Dignity law. I unconditionally support that. When it comes to persons with dementia who want to die, they need to be able to be very clear about what their intentions are and why."

John exclaimed, "But starvation and dehydration look like a punishment, and they really feel like a punishment. There's nothing we can do for Dan but wait until he gets worse. It is terribly unpleasant for him and for the people around him."

I was curious and asked John, "If Dan could speak at this point, what would he say about VSED?"

The gist of John's reply was that Dan would have stated his preference to take the overdose and gotten everything done and over with quickly. But his shift to VSED was engendered by the hope that family members would *not* consider it to be in the same realm as suicide. This proved to mostly be the case, as it settled the concerns of some family members. But unfortunately, not all of them were mollified.

"We were a little naive about how people would respond to announcing the date he chose," John acknowledged. "So, VSED has eased people into the reality of Dan's death. I guess it would be safe to say we wish everyone had had the response to our plan to ingest pharmaceuticals that we wanted them to have. But they didn't. Obviously, everybody is suffering. I don't mean to sound like there is anyone who isn't. But I think VSED—if *easier* is a word you can use in this context—is *easier* for the Winter family. However, it's not *easier* for Dan."

"Pardon an innocent question," I said. "But I just need you to put something into words. Tell me, in what manner is Dan suffering?"

"He's not had any interest in food for many days," John said, "so that's less of a concern. However, thirst has been constant. The pain from his headaches has been intense. When he's awake, it's clear from the expression on his face that something is hurting him all the time. I don't know what it's like to have not eaten or had anything to drink for 7 to 10 days. I don't know what he would say if he were able."

*****

The following day, John and I spoke briefly, but there wasn't a lot more to report. Dan was now completely incapable of talking. He mainly slept. Friday lay on the bed with him. John monitored things, tried to keep busy, and periodically administered morphine.

On the day before Dan's death, his mother and younger sister called the apartment. According to John, "They asked if I would put the phone up to his ear, so they could say goodbye.... He had been sleeping soundly, but when he heard his mother's voice, he woke up, put his hand over my hand, which was holding the phone, and tried to talk. He made sounds but didn't say any words. He seemed to recognize his mother's and sister's voices. After the call ended, he closed his eyes. It was the last time he tried to communicate."

"It's remarkable," I said. "When you think that the first experience one has as we come into this world is emerging from our mother's womb and perhaps being placed on her breast.... And then to go out with her voice in your ear? Astonishing!"

"Yeah," said John. "It's maybe too romantic an idea to believe. But that's what happened."

John went on to say that a friend came over and sat at the bedside with him. Dan's breathing began to noticeably change in the late afternoon—it got irregular, shallower, and then a persistent rattle could be heard.

During those last couple of nights, Friday had commenced a new series of behaviors: around 4 AM each morning, she would get agitated, stand up, and walk back and forth in the bed between Dan and his spouse. The dog would then scoot up close to her master, a few inches from his face, and stare silently. John couldn't determine whether she was smelling Dan's breath or just looking into his closed eyes, but she would do that for 15 minutes while not moving a hair. John found it impossible to sleep and retreated into another room.

Early in the morning of day 13, John momentarily fell asleep in front of the television. Upon awakening, he entered the bedroom to check on his spouse. He observed that Friday was maintaining her vigil, but Dan had stopped breathing.

"There was still some warmth," John told me. "He hadn't been dead all that long, but I checked his pulse and...."

I broke in and asked, "He had quietly died?"

"Yup. Absolutely," John murmured. He then added, as an afterthought, "Dan had not budged from the same position that he was in all of Tuesday."

John called the hospice, which promptly and efficiently dealt with the death certification and other matters. His next phone call was to Dan's mother. "She wasn't terribly surprised because of the conversation they'd had the day before," he said. "She spent most of the time consoling me, which was sweet and generous." John was crying softly when he said, "How can a mother find time to do anything like that after she has just lost a child—a son? It meant a lot to me."

The next call was to Oregon Health and Science University for the body donation. John explained: "Friday hadn't left Dan's side after he died, but when the staff person came to get his body that morning, she was on high alert. She didn't bark, but she was staring quizzically at the people. There was a kind of anxious intensity that I don't remember seeing her exhibit previously, and she got up and followed them as they took Dan out on the gurney to the door and to the elevator. . . . I then fed and took her for a walk."

He continued: "On every other day, Friday ran to find Dan upon returning home. On this day, she didn't. She did not look for him. Her focus was on me, her next nap, and, of course, her next meal. She seemed to understand that Dan was gone. Really gone."

Later that night, Friday climbed into bed and rested her head upon Dan's pillow. She focused her big, chocolate-colored eyes on John, until she finally fell asleep. She had established a new nightly routine.

*****

Dan had asked John to post an email after his death. John began it with an introduction, which read as follows:

> *Dan died on February 3, 2021. He wanted this letter sent out on the day he died, but I'm getting to it now. This may come as a shock to some of you, and for others it's a message you've anticipated. Do feel free to write or email or text me. I intend to save all the comments I get to give to his three children. I, too, thank you for your love and friendship. . . . He leaves a big hole in many hearts . . . .*

The email composed by Dan then continued:

> *To my Friends and Family members,*
>
> *Many of you know that I've been living with early-onset Alzheimer's disease since my diagnosis in December 2017. You may also know that I've remained steadfast in my plan to take my own life before the disease, inevitably, takes away my agency and my free will.*
>
> *I'm ending my lucky and love-filled life today, at age 62, in the Portland home that John and I share with our fantastic labradoodle, Friday, both of whom have been my constant companions in this decline, this theft of identity. The decision to control how I die has been a source of great comfort to*

me as my symptoms have quickened in their capacity to remind me that I'm losing myself to the disease in an unrelenting fashion that defies description.

To be sure, I've had more than several conversations with loving, well-meaning people who have strenuously objected to my end-of-life plan. But, this decision can't be made by committee. It's all on me. I've lived a charmed life.

The pain I feel as I prepare to leave all of you has at times been crippling. And, it's been John Forsgren, my dear husband, who has kept me going fueled by gratitude, humor, grace, and a sense of simple elegance in his daily life that rubs off on most everything he does.

I wish we were talking in person so I could tell you how much you have meant to me. I am so grateful you were part of my life. Simply put, I'm a guy who became better because of my relationship with you.

With love,

Dan

28

After Dan's death I continued to call John, first every 2 weeks, and then monthly, and then every 6 weeks. All the while, I worked on the manuscript. Our subsequent interviews took place over the next 3 years. During that time, I, too, was mourning Dan. Frankly, it was helpful for me to learn about the details of John's deeper and infinitely more intense bereavement experience. In addition, our conversations provided an opportunity to fact-check the events of the 9 months that had led up to his death and, in some instances, to observe how they could take on a different meaning with the passage of time.

The sweet romance between the two men touched me, and I felt myself pulled along in John's wake as he dealt with grief. I envied him his emotional awareness, resilience, and the support provided by his extensive friendship network—his logical family. It was humbling to see how these connections sustained John.

One week after Dan's death, I began our interview by asking, "How are you holding up?"

He answered, "It's getting harder every day. There are things that need to get done, and I'm finding it difficult to generate the necessary energy. I have been told to give myself permission to do things at my own speed—and I will. I have been in touch with a few friends. People have dropped off food for me in the lobby of the building, and that's been nice. One friend made soup, and she wanted to bring it directly to me. This was the day before yesterday. She walked in, and we stepped away from each other, and then we just kind of fell into each other's arms. It was the first hug I had received since Dan died. It made me realize the importance of hugs. For the last 2 nights, I've had dinner with neighbors. I'm glad they're all within my bubble, so that I can eat inside with a mask off and feel reasonably safe."

John talked about some recordings that had recently been made by Dan's brother-in-law. He was unsure about when he'd want to listen to them but recalled that his own father wrote a memoir and had also made audio recordings. This took place when his parents and younger sister were in Vietnam. "My father did the recordings back in 1974," said John, "to send to his partners in their Oregon medical clinic. Shortly after his death, one of those business partners forwarded them to me, and it was an impactful experience to hear his voice again."

"In addition," he continued, "I recorded a couple of conversations with my mother during her dementia to get a sense of what she recalled. The memories about her childhood and young adulthood were very intact. It was really fun to listen to her talk about that part of her life."

"Dementia?" I asked. "What dementia?" This was the first time John mentioned to me that his mother had a dementia.

It turned out that, when she was 76, his mother was diagnosed with metastatic breast cancer and simultaneously began having a series of small strokes. They affected her coordination and led to a multi-infarct, vascular dementia.

On one occasion while assisting her with toileting, she looked John in the eye and said, "Did you ever think that you'd be wiping your mother's ass?"

This reminded me of the book, *Tuesdays with Morrie*, where the amiable protagonist, who has amyotrophic lateral sclerosis (ALS), announces early on that he'd prefer to die if he ever reaches the point of no longer being able to wipe his own buttocks.[1] Interestingly, that time comes and goes, and Morrie takes no action to shorten his life.

John told me it was probably the first and only time he ever heard his mother use that word.

During the last 3 years of life, her short-term memory was distinctly impaired, and she had occasional hallucinations. She was regularly receiving treatment for the breast cancer when John suddenly recalled that his mother had always told the family she was opposed to such life-prolonging therapies. As a nurse, she had witnessed plenty of instances when medical care was counterproductive.

"So, one day," John said, "I inquired of my sister, 'Why is Mom still getting cancer treatment?' Until then nobody had thought to ask." His sister, Beth, then brought this up with their mother, who declared, "Of course, we should stop the treatment." The chemotherapy was discontinued, and, 4 months afterward, she peacefully died.

"The obvious question," I asked, "is to what extent did your mother's illnesses and her death influence your response to Dan's dementia and his death?

John paused only briefly before replying that having had a father who was a physician and a mother who was a nurse, both parents were always upfront about symptoms, diagnoses, and treatment. They each appreciated the limitations of modern medicine and spoke about this frequently. In his family, death

---

[1] Albom Mitch. *Tuesdays with Morrie: An Old Man, a Young Man, and Life's Greatest Lesson*, 25th *Anniversary Edition* (New York: Crown Publishing Group, 2002).

was considered a natural phenomenon. His parents consistently maintained that there was no shame in either contracting an illness or of dying; individuals should have the right to determine their own terminal preferences.

I'm not sure if John directly answered my question about the impact of his mother's dementia and death on his response to Dan's illness, but I think he was well primed to respond empathically to that situation.

After a pause, he then continued: "Keep in mind that I had been dealing with HIV for 20 years before my parents began to face their own end-of-life choices. While watching them die was difficult because I loved them, it didn't have the kind of rawness that occurred back in 1989, when I sat down and began a list of gay friends who had died from AIDS. I stopped at 100."

After we hung up, I kept thinking: *John stopped at 100? What does the immensity of that do to a person?*

*****

As we reviewed the circumstances preceding Dan's death, John recalled the late summer and fall as having been a period in which his husband was mentally preparing to die. At no point did Dan subscribe to Simon and Garfunkel's lyrics: "So, I'll continue to continue to pretend, my life will never end, and flowers never bend, with the rainfall."[2] Despite or perhaps because of the imminence of death, the two of them were, according to John, "still having a wonderful time together enjoying the normalcy of our very unobtrusive, simple lives of cooking, walking the dog, watching television, and dull, dull, dull stuff that Dan really relished."

It was just a few weeks before Christmas when Dan "lost track of himself while walking Friday in the park." That was a crucial indicator of the disease deteriorating into an entirely unacceptable category, and the serious planning began in earnest to truncate the illness.

Despite the ensuing drama, John remained convinced, "If I were to create a how-to-list, it would include a step of telling one's family that you will be setting a date. 'Yes,' I would say, 'the actual date of death will be determined between now and when I send out the final date.' I would really want family members to be prepared. Of course, every family is going to be different, and people need to anticipate that there could be some sizeable bumps.

"VSED is a pretty rough way to die," John decided, "and Dan was lucky it took only 13 days. In that time, he lost nearly 30 pounds. However, he was ready for the fast to go on considerably longer."

---

[2] Simon and Garfunkel, "Flowers never bend with the rainfall," Genius.com, accessed November 18, 2022, https://genius.com/Simon-and-garfunkel-flowers-never-bend-with-the-rainfall-lyrics.

John appreciated that, in deep clinical depressions, people feel despairing, isolated, helpless, and hopeless, and they *should* receive aggressive efforts to keep them from ending their own lives. But he insisted this was never Dan's situation, and there are plenty of folk, like his husband, who ought to have access to a variety of different means to bring their lives to a close. "We're asking," said John, "for our life's boundaries to be thoughtfully considered and not just circumscribed by some ancient idea of what suicide means and what constitutes sin. Just because others haven't caught on, there's no reason to disbelieve what I know to be true: people should have the right to control the conclusion of life."

*****

A couple of weeks later, John slipped into a period of numbness in which he could not bear to speak about anything related to Dan. Grief formed an impenetrable barrier between him and the rest of the world, and he found himself uninterested in the daily newspaper and its headlines. The labradoodle became more important than ever in helping to shape his daily activities. He told me, "Friday lost her master and is now entirely dependent on me. I must get up to feed her and take her out for her morning walk *or there will be consequences*. And, I'd rather not have to clean up those consequences."

"People do come to appreciate their pets more at such moments," I suggested. It was one of those polite and banal comments I regret occasionally making.

But John blew past it. "Yup," he exclaimed and took a deep, shuddering breath. "There were several days when I was crying much of the time—especially when I talked to people on the phone—and then she would jump up on my lap. If I cried, there would be a light clatter of nails on the polished hardwood floors. Then she'd appear as if by magic and stare into my face the way she did when Dan was asleep. She can recognize when either of us is hurting, and her inclination is to get as close as possible to offer succor."

He went on, "Like any dog that's well loved, she's a powerful life force. Plus, she's a constant reminder to me of Dan and the relationship they had together."

Upon reflection, when I had first tried to compose an essay about Dan's death, I found that I wrote it largely from Friday's perspective. I was struck by her appreciation of his decline and wish to be with him. It seemed that the dog was now trying to sustain John through a difficult phase of mourning.

"There were times," John explained, "when Dan would travel and take Friday with him to Missoula or on road trips to Kansas City. I would be keenly aware of the cold emptiness when both Dan and Friday were gone. Currently there is this enormous void from Dan's death, but with Friday around, it's not entirely cold. There's always some warmth."

*****

When we spoke in March, John had just gotten vaccinated and felt like he could think again about the possibility of future travel. "Potent" was the word he used to describe this step, and John went on to say, "friends are helping me with all the decisions that need to be made. I understand now better than before how important it is to not make big judgments while grieving. But some must be made, and fortunately, I have this small army of friends who are stepping forward to give meaningful help."

One of these friends, he explained, was encouraging him to join her on regular walks; another provided financial advice; another cooked and shared meals. "Yet I am constantly aware of how easy it would be right now to slip into a depression," he said. "For all of the horrors, it's such a comfortable and embracing place to be.

"Lew," he said, "dealing with reality is hard."

I agreed but remained silent.

He went on: "It may be surprising, but I am grateful for having had the experience of a major depression in 2009–2010, from which I recovered. The tools to manage depression are simple, although they're not always easy to follow. But so far, I have been accomplishing what is required to a very large degree."

"Given how Dan died, have you been thinking about taking your own life?" I asked. Perhaps I was channeling the man from Kansas, but I felt like my relationship allowed me to explore any and all topics.

"I have no desire to die," John replied. "I still don't know what the future holds, but these last 10 years with Dan really awakened me to so many of the good things that can happen in life . . . things that really had seemed remote in the months before I met him, back when I was depressed."

John proceeded to weave together his thoughts about opposition to the Vietnam war, his role in the gay rights movement, experience as an AIDS activist, and his current position about the right to die. "In order to change things," he told me, "it takes real passion. It requires an earnest commitment to an idea, and it requires creating a community. Dan and I were aware from the very beginning that taking his life after being diagnosed with dementia was a very personal act. It was also a political act. We obviously knew that we were going up against the cultural norm and there would be backlash."

John continued, "I was just reading through one of Dan's notebooks. It's not really a diary, but it has references to things he did and to his observations. At the end of one entry, he wrote, 'I am resolute.' And because that's all I ever saw from him; I wasn't surprised to read it. But I was moved by his having written those three words down, knowing that when you write something, it is different than just thinking it. Yes, there was nothing in any of those pages in which he questioned whether he was about to do the right thing. He was genuinely resolute."

John vividly recalls his first trip to Kansas, where he witnessed how dementia had ravaged Dan's father. "We both reacted the same way," he said. "You should have a right to take control over parts of our lives that the culture has traditionally said, 'No, you don't.' The visit only reinforced what both of us strongly felt to be true. So, when Dan got his diagnosis there was never a question of what he would do. The act merged intellectual, emotional, and political convictions."

*****

John made dinner for the couple who lived next door and who had primarily fed him while Dan was not eating and drinking. He found it was simply wonderful to spend a day composing a menu, shopping, and cooking and then having people join him at his dining room table. It felt normal. A few days later, he did the same thing for the two men who invited him to join them for their nightly routine, including cocktails. One evening, he went to a restaurant with yet another friend, and they comfortably sat outside to dine. He felt like life was edging back to a semblance of normal.

But he was also forging a deeper realization that Dan was gone *forever*. The intense awareness, the calamitous grief, would sometimes paralyze him. One day, it produced an intense pain that left him breathless. "What went through my head at that instant was, *He's really gone!* The silly, simple realization washed over me. I continue to have experiences all day, every day, where I think of something that I want to tell him—all the usual grief things. I'm continuing to try to talk to friends at least once every day. But I failed to do that twice last week. Instead, I kind of curled up and didn't leave the condo. I began to cry. Then I heard a bark, and Friday jumped up into my arms."

John keened, "I miss him. I just miss him. I miss him. I miss him. It's not much more complicated."

"Grief comes in waves, the classic pangs of grief," the psychiatrist, Dr. Madeline Li, wrote in an essay. "I know it will take time, but it is a timeless moment. I have been struck by how many of my emotional moments come on abruptly, seemingly disconnected from thoughts of my mother, as if my grief is an autonomous process."[3]

A journalist similarly and succinctly observed, "the ordinariness of grief governs my days."[4]

[3] Madeline Li, "Daughter, doctor, death broker: A MAiD provider in her mother's last days," Maclean's, accessed September 29, 2022, https://www.macleans.ca/society/daughter-doctor-death-broker-a-maid-provider-in-her-mothers-last-days/.

[4] Margaret Renkl, "More and more, I talk to the dead," *The New York Times*, accessed January 31, 2023, https://www.nytimes.com/2023/01/30/opinion/death-grief-memory.html.

During the interview, John's mood abruptly changed, and he observed, "The weather has been really beautiful." Earlier in the day, the widower had sat down with a friend in her garden and noted that "the cherry trees were blooming like crazy, and the blossoms were fluttering and falling like snow." He said to me, "I was pleased to be with my friend. I needed to be with somebody." The two of them sat together on a bench in the picturesque backyard while talking about their feelings and how to resist allowing themselves to become isolated.

Since 2004, John had been a member of a book club that was scheduled to have its next virtual meeting later in the week. It had been John's turn to pick a book, and he impulsively selected *Catcher in the Rye*.[5] After he finished reading it, John wondered, *Why in the world do they teach that in high school?* The story seemed to be so much more sophisticated than what he recalled.

Then he flashed back to attending a Zoom meeting of the book club in October when Dan was struggling over selecting a date to end his life. At the time, John was listening carefully to the lively literary discussion on the computer, when, "I suddenly had to leave. I just had to go and sit down with Dan." He signed off, and "that was the last I tried to participate in the book club. The time spent together with Dan had just become so much more intense and valuable to me."

I mused, *When John next rejoins his group, we'll have to see how it goes with Holden Caulfield.* I thought it interesting that he had selected this J. D. Salinger novel, which features a 16-year-old protagonist calling out society's foibles and proclaiming, "I'm always saying 'Glad to've met you' to someone I'm not at all glad I met. If you want to stay alive, you have to say that stuff, though." Part of what I think John was experiencing was the realization that at certain points in bereavement, one needs to just go through the motions. You may not sincerely feel like doing some things or engaging with other people, but it is restorative to continue trying.

[5] J. D. Salinger, *Catcher in the Rye* (New York: Little, Brown and Company, 1951).

29

John busied himself appraising and packing away Dan's collection of mid-century and contemporary regional art. According to the will, John was responsible for its dispersal, and Dan's family members had the right of first refusal. Accordingly, they needed to know the cost of each piece. Fortunately, before his death, Dan had deaccessioned and auctioned many of the most valuable works. But what remained was still an onerous task, and one that required considerable effort and diplomacy.

"I've given a lot of thought about Dan's role in the family," John said. "He would have been the first to declare that he was an imperfect man. But he was the heart of the extended clan—except for his beloved mother. Dan was the uncle that the nieces and nephews chose to hang out with, and he was the relative they wanted to visit. He infused the family with a kind and gentle energy, and he nurtured them. I think the Winters will have to go through a period of considerable adjustment to find a substitute for Dan."

John continued, "He was different from the others because he had dealt with really difficult personal issues, like sexual abuse, alcoholism, being gay, and finally, having a degenerative illness. He was different in that he had lost the fear of talking about problematic things."

I realized, as John spoke, it was exactly this quality that impressed me in the very first minutes when I met Dan and just how much I appreciate his unabashed earnestness. Psychiatrists from my generation are accustomed to remaining neutral, echoing people's statements with a question mark attached, and rarely revealing our backgrounds or personal reactions. Honesty is one of my core values, but I prefer to remain in the background—unlike Dan's eagerness to provoke, instruct, invite, and entertain. I grinned as I thought about him joyfully singing, dancing, and whisking a bowl of eggs to a Whitney Houston song while making breakfast for his family!

I could easily imagine his influence on the younger members of the clan. To them, he must have been an incredibly zany, loving uncle—the guy who broke with the norms, could listen in a nonjudgmental manner, and was equally liable to say almost anything in response. He was a fearless, outrageous, and yet vulnerable older man who identified with outcasts and outlaws, who lived well but worried about those without homes, and who devoted himself to a host of other social justice causes. He was their uncle, who had been through hell but was still unquestionably a loyal Winter. His early life may have been marked by concealment and secrecy, but as a middle-aged man Dan acquired a certain rectitude and had become—dare I say—righteous. At the same time, he was an iconoclast who rejected Alzheimer's ordinary course and was determined to end his life.

There were additional questions on my mind of the kind that polite people don't articulate, but ones that, nevertheless, I wished to ask the bereaved spouse. "How do you feel about the way Dan chose to die?" I found myself inquiring. "Would it have been better if he had taken the overdose as he fully intended? Should he have kept quiet about the date, anticipating that some of the family were going to react badly? We've touched on these matters before, but what do you think about them today?"

"Ahh, hindsight," he muttered. "Dan and I both believed that this subject needs to be broached. We should all be willing to talk to our beloveds about what it is we want at the end of our lives and what kind of control we wish to maintain. I've thought about what would have happened if we hadn't announced anything before the 15th of January and Dan took the overdose and I then notified the family. It would have been a more graceful exit. But I think that his certainty about wanting control prevented him from acting in a way that could have been interpreted as shameful. . . . Dan didn't want anybody to think he was ashamed of what he was doing. Secrecy would have had its benefits, but it might've been more difficult for me to convince people that Dan hadn't been regretful. He wanted people to know because he told them."

"So, you're telling me that silence would have been out of character?"

"Yup."

"He had to explicitly state what he was going to do," I suggested. "He had to say when he was going to do it, even though in hindsight it was a mistake?"

"Well, I'm not willing to say that it was a mistake. When we talked about Dan's Alzheimer's and how he intended to take control of the end of his life, it was always political as well as intensely personal. He wasn't starting a movement; however, politics had always been a part of his life, whether it was Planned Parenthood or the ACLU or when he created a team of young Black boys from challenged Kansas City neighborhoods and introduced them to the world of organized basketball. He enjoyed the kids individually, but it was also a political action that he was performing. When it came to how he was going to die, we always talked about this as being a political act. We discussed how you're invariably going to alienate some people; other folk are just going to shrug their shoulders; and still others are going to think about ending their own lives in different ways. The last was always Dan's special hope."

John said, "Not that they would make the choice he made, but they would make a decision for themselves after considering the various options."

"And they would consider the options to include an overdose or to stop eating and drinking?" I inquired.

"Or the option of letting the disease control their fate," John said. "He and I would never try to talk somebody out of the idea of letting Alzheimer's do its thing. There are people who think, *Gee whiz! Grandma seems really happy staring out her window or watching television all day long.* Well, so be it!"

I said to John, "One of the things I spoke to Dan about—unfortunately very late in the game when he was having trouble stringing thoughts together—was also clearly a political thing. It had to do with MAiD [medical assistance in dying] laws and how they exclude, at least in this country, people who have dementing illnesses. What I thought I heard him saying—and I just want to check it out with you—was this was something he felt was wrong and something he hoped would change."

"That's entirely true. It's what I mean by a political act. What Dan did and what the end-of-life movement is all about remains a concept that is still alien to many people. The public is more comfortable *not* discussing it and much more comfortable being angry or upset even when somebody merely thinks about it. What Dan did, well, it needs to be put into words. If you don't find language to describe the behavior, then it becomes a very difficult thing to actually consider."

At that instant the word that came to my mind was "taboo." Defined as being something that is not acceptable to say, mention, or do, Dan clearly transgressed a deeply rooted societal taboo. Shortly afterward I wasn't surprised to hear about the disintegration of a short-lived formal agreement between Compassion & Choices (C&C) and the Alzheimer's Association. The two nonprofits had planned on providing education between their members, but when this became more widely known, the agreement fell apart.[1,2] The Alzheimer's Association, which encourages its members to hope for cures and contribute to cutting-edge research, issued an apologetic statement saying that it had "failed to do

[1] Luis Miguel, "Exposed: Alzheimer's org frantically cuts ties with assisted suicide group," *New American*, accessed February 1, 2023, https://thenewamerican.com/exposed-alzheimers-org-frantically-cuts-ties-with-assisted-suicide-group/.

[2] Alexander Raikin, "Alzheimer's Association hides new partnership with lobbying group for assisted suicide," *The Washington Free Beacon*, accessed January 30, 2023, https://freebeacon.com/policy/alzheimers-association-hides-new-partnership-with-lobbying-group-for-assisted-suicide/?_ga=2.63147311.1085654935.1675173828-1065187458.1675173828.

appropriate due diligence" when it collaborated with C&C[3] The organization's spokesperson went on to announce that C&C's values "are inconsistent with those of the Association. We deeply regret our mistake, have begun the termination of the relationship, and apologize to all of the families we support who were hurt or disappointed."

Yes. Definitely a taboo.

John continued: "While it would have been nice if Dan's family had responded to his announcement with a single voice of support, what actually happened reflects social reality. It is how *most* Americans, *most* people, at this moment in time, think about these choices. *They are conflicted.* I don't know how you're going to describe it in the book, but Dan made use of VSED hoping it might *soften* the reaction of the people in his family who reflexively objected. I think that's an important story to tell."

"Yes," I said.

I thought of the journalist, Laurie Loisel, currently Director of Communication and Outreach, Northwestern District Attorney's Office in Massachusetts, who wrote me (January 31, 2023, email): "Had I known about VSED when my 82-year-old father died the way he told us he intended to, in a police station parking lot, using a gun he had purchased without our knowledge, I would have suggested it. I believe VSED should be an active option on the table for anyone nearing the end of life or looking to have some agency around the dying process. This process fills the gap where the medical aid in dying option is not available: for people who have no immediate terminal diagnosis, but for whom the next chapter they face is simply unacceptable. I believe people have the right to make those decisions for themselves. It seems completely in keeping with hospice philosophy to accept people who exercise this option into their care; in fact, I'd say it seems inhumane not to."[4]

However, John, reflecting on Dan's relatively drawn-out death, then asked me: "Is starving oneself to death better than using pharmaceuticals? Is it different from suicide? I think these need to be considered carefully. Is the punishment that comes with depriving oneself of food and water somehow less sinful, less onerous, less evil, less . . . whatever it is that's in people's minds? I don't know."

He went on to say: "VSED is a readily available death-accelerating method for people with dementia or those who are seeking a nontechnological death. But I think we need to look at it, hopefully, as a temporary, short-term answer to the

---

[3] "Alzheimer's Association Statement About Compassion & Choices," Alzheimer's Association, accessed February 1, 2023, https://www.alz.org/news/2023/alzheimers-association-statement?_ga=2.60548397.1085654935.1675173828-1065187458.1675173828.

[4] Laurie Loisel, *On Their Own Terms: How One Woman's Choice to Die Helped Me Understand My Father's Suicide* (Amherst, MA: Levellers Press, 2019).

problem of those who want to die. The long-term answer is that we need to offer other quieter, more peaceful, faster, and legal means to die."

John's remarks reminded me of comments by the retired National Public Radio talk show host, Diane Rehm, whose husband made use of VSED to end his many years of decline from progressive Parkinson's disease. It took 10 days for him to die, and Ms. Rehm described his death as "excruciating to witness."[5] She later said in a film based on her experience as a caregiver, "Each of us is just one bad death away from supporting these [MAiD] laws."[6]

As we spoke, I felt myself getting riled up and asked John, "What I heard from Dan—and what I think that I'm hearing from you—is we should institute new laws that modify the existing statutes?"

"I understand," he said, "why the American right-to-die organizations have taken an incremental approach toward drafting laws. I understand why when it comes to dementia their present focus is on advance directives which say, 'Stop feeding me and stop giving me liquids when I no longer recognize my children and have ceased eating on my own.' However, I think it is time that people with Alzheimer's can be educated to take advantage of a DIY suicide or to have laws—like those in several Western European countries—that allow compassionate medical staff to actively assist in putting an end to the lives of suffering individuals who have dementias and chronic disorders."

But it is still the rare palliative medicine provider, like Dr. Jeffrey A. Zesiger (February 3, 2023, email), Medical Director at Hospice of the Fisher Home, who is unafraid to state: "When a person with a terminal illness—and Alzheimer's disease falls into that category in my opinion—chooses to forgo treatment or seeks MAiD or undergoes VSED, I respect them. It is their life, not mine. It is the quality of life that is the yardstick for each of us. If the quality of life is poor at the end, I believe we should listen and allow our patients to die sooner, compassionately, and with professional support. Otherwise, it is we who cause their suffering or force them to contemplate harsh ways to die."

I was still uncomfortable writing about the negative reaction among Dan's relatives, and I turned to John for advice. "You must avoid whitewashing this topic," he stated emphatically, "because the majority of American families *will* have a hard time with this whole thing. Dan and I certainly hoped it wouldn't happen. We talked about it and took every step we could think of to prepare them for this. We learned that even the best laid plans can't sometimes overcome fear and ignorance. The politics of the issue scream out that some family

[5] Jane E. Brody, "When patients choose to end their lives: For some, the decision to die is more complicated than a wish to reduce pain," *The New York Times*, accessed May 18, 2023, https://www.nytimes.com/2021/04/05/well/live/aid-in-dying.html.

[6] "When My Time Comes," https://whenmytimecomesmovie.com/.

opposition will almost inevitably occur, but that doesn't mean we shouldn't go ahead. It only means that we should anticipate these reactions, make our plans, and create laws that empower the individual—regardless of whether the family has reached a consensus to support him or her."

The patient's right to privacy is spelled out in Canada's Criminal Code, and it allows eligible individuals who pursue MAiD to stipulate whether others should be informed. This may not please everyone. It did not please Cheryl Hiebert's family.

Cheryl Hiebert was a Canadian woman with early-onset Alzheimer's who applied for and received a medically assisted death but did not inform any of her kin.[7] Her sister, Cynthia Hiebert, was later quoted as saying that because of Cheryl's decision, "we all feel like something was ripped away from us, and we want that goodbye. We want that closure."

With no details about a cause of death, the Hiebert family spent the first few days baffled and desperate to find out what happened. A subsequent investigation by the Office of the Chief Coroner concluded that the usual procedures for MAiD were followed, and Hiebert was deemed competent to have made informed healthcare-related decisions. The report did *not* raise concerns of coercion or undue influence.

A lawyer representing Hiebert's estate later provided documents, including a series of letters signed by her. One of these was entitled, "Why I Didn't Tell You."

"This is really hard to write," it reads. "I have always known since the day I was told that I had young-onset dementia, Alzheimer's type, that I would pursue medical assistance in dying. I have lived with that for years and I recognize that you haven't. The fact that I didn't tell you doesn't mean that I don't love you. I do love you and I know that you love me. . . ."

She wrote in another missive, "I watched my mother fade away with this disease. She deteriorated and had to go into long-term care. . . . I don't want to go to long-term care. It is not a quality of life. I want a meaningful life. I want purpose and involvement and conversation."

But these letters and documents have not satisfied her sister, Cynthia, who a year later explains: "I'm so angry because you cannot heal. It's still haunting me. . . ."

There is no correct answer, but Dan's and Cheryl Hiebert's experiences suggest that some family members and friends are bound to be distressed whether or not one informs loved ones about the means and timing to hasten death. It

---

[7] Brandie Weikle and Brian Goldman, "This family learned loved one had medically assisted death only after she was gone: Patients have a right to privacy on this matter, says Ontario's chief coroner," CBC Radio, accessed October 13, 2022, https://www.cbc.ca/radio/whitecoat/this-family-learned-loved-one-had-medically-assisted-death-only-after-she-was-gone-1.6380470.

is the truly fortunate and probably unusual family where everyone is on the same page.

*****

A memorial event was held in Kansas City and attended by several of Dan's family; it included more than 100 people who gathered to raise money for ACLU internships in his name. John was pleased to hear about it, but the pandemic foreclosed any possible desire on his part to travel and join them.

"There have been some long, dark days," John told me. "I have been missing him so deeply. The shock has worn off. I can feel myself moving out of the life that we shared into my new life of being alone. I'm experiencing what I read happens all the time—that when you begin to make changes because the other person isn't there, you wonder, Am I going to forget? Am I being disloyal? Am I. . . . There are a lot of pretty irrational thoughts. But nevertheless, they are not keeping me from doing things. I don't wish to succumb to the fear of changing or to the anxiety of moving on. Nor do I feel like I have a timeline."

I listened and thought, *Grief and relief make for peculiar bedfellows.*

John said: "I may be belaboring the point, but I had wanted to do some work at home, because I've completely moved out of the studio. I got a couple of 5-foot-long stainless steel tables, and this afternoon I'm going to start preparing new canvases and begin working on some pieces."

He continued, "I have got to do this because of Dan. He would want me to make art in our home. I used to show him everything I did, and his delight and satisfaction were really important to me."

30

John resumed feeling more creative, energetic, and even playful; but the man's grief pervaded our interviews. Being an artist, he was cursed by residual images burned into his brain that could not be easily ablated. Prominent among these was the rictus of terror on Dan's face after getting lost with Friday at the park. John sought to resolve any ill feelings on his part prompted by the dissension that had erupted within the Winter family around Dan's death.[1] As more and more time passed and the pandemic lessened in intensity, John powerfully connected with his logical family and began to feel as if normality was returning.

We remained in regular contact, and John sent me a brief excerpt from one of Dan's notebooks written shortly after the diagnosis: "I have no intention of letting my disease take its own course without interruption. I will not grow into a shell of a person, just simply breathing but having no executive functioning, no memory, no compassion, empathy, choice, or sense of humor or even any sense of self. It was extraordinary to see my dad in that state—remarkably dispiriting. I do not intend to have my most loved ones suffer watching me."[2]

Dan's words reminded me of Susan Sontag's description of cancer, which can equally apply to AIDS and to Alzheimer's: it is "an evil, invincible predator, not just a disease."[3] In all three of these illnesses a beloved person slowly disappears in front of your eyes. The notebook affirmed for John that Dan intended to die not only to avoid the deterioration of the disorder but to also spare him and the Winter family from having to witness that decline.

*****

[1] Catherine Pearson, "The emotional relief of forgiving someone," *The New York Times*. accessed January 26, 2023, https://www.nytimes.com/2023/04/28/well/forgiveness-mental-health.html.

[2] D. Winter, "Entry from January 15, 2018," in *Dan Winter's Diary*.

[3] Susan Sontag Foundation, "Illness as metaphor and AIDS and its metaphors," accessed September 10, 2023, http://www.susansontag.com/SusanSontag/books/illnessAsMetaphorExce rpt.shtml.

As the writing project reached its final stage, I wanted to answer the question for myself as to whether Dan had a "good death."

My psychiatric mentors, Drs. Avery D. Weisman (d. January 2, 2017) and Thomas Hackett (d. January 23, 1988) approached the question of a good death by wisely recognizing that although the medical profession is dedicated to survival and health, it cannot indefinitely postpone dying. Half a century ago, they observed, "people's attitudes toward death correspond to their attitudes toward life; how each person dies is determined by how he has lived."[4,5] The two scholars—one a renowned psychoanalyst and the other the celebrated chair of psychiatry at the Massachusetts General Hospital—were revolutionary in opining that it can be appropriate and not necessarily psychopathological for the tormented and/or the imminently dying to want to abbreviate life. In their writings, they took the position that death is often a positive solution rather than a catastrophe. In stating such a position, they made it explicit that not all voluntary deaths are either cruel, unthinkable, destructive, or unacceptable. I am especially a great fan of their concise definition of a good death as being "the type of death one would choose if there were a choice."

So, how might this pertain to Dan and to dementia?

Most individuals have given little thought to the possibility that they may receive this diagnosis. It is a disconcerting, terrifying, but vague possibility, and even if they have witnessed friends or family with Alzheimer's disease, humans are programmed to *not* believe that they will have to endure this misfortune themselves. We are an optimistic species. But while people would like to live to 90 or older, they cannot usually grasp that the odds are 1 in 3 that they will have developed a dementia.[6] That's 1 in 3! However, despite this, relatively few men and women complete advance directives—let alone, dementia directives—and even when people appoint healthcare proxies, they only rarely provide them with explicit instructions about what they would want under such circumstances.

Between overcoming his life's challenges and witnessing the last phase of his father's life, Dan managed to acquire the necessary fortitude to confront Alzheimer's. The first two-thirds of his life may have demanded secrecy, but in his last years he was determined to make amends and act differently. One result was his insistence on openly and honestly communicating exactly how he

[4] Lewis M. Cohen, *A Dignified Ending: Taking Control Over How We Die* (Lanham, MD: Rowman & Littlefield, 2019), 50.

[5] A. D. Weisman and T. P. Hackett, "Predilection to death: Death and dying as a psychiatric problem," *Psychosomatic Medicine* 23 (1961): 232–256. PMID: 13784028.

[6] "Fact Sheet: U.S. Dementia Trends," PRB, October 21, 2021, https://www.prb.org/resources/fact-sheet-u-s-dementia-trends/#:~:text=Dementia%20is%20more%20prevalent%20at,adults%20ages%2090%20and%20older.

intended to behave. He knew that such a campaign wouldn't necessarily help his family to reach a consensus—but that didn't stop him from trying.

From his many years directing the ACLU of Kansas and Western Missouri, Dan understood that we inhabit a messy, contradictory world. He appreciated that human beings are programmed to have "cognitive biases that nudge us toward self-congratulatory narratives in which our own side is virtuously battling idiots on the other side."[7] But his tumultuous life allowed him to acquire an unusual degree of balance and maturity. He could be confident in his opinions and desires while simultaneously accepting that others would differ.

During the final months, he wanted—given the restrictions of COVID and the limitations of his Alzheimer's symptoms—to spend as much time as possible with John and his nuclear family. He kept his husband apprised about every step of his journey, and Dan also protected him from having to make those tough decisions. He explicitly trusted John to be his faithful ally.

Throughout the time that I knew him, Dan was absolutely committed to having both an authentic life *and* death while not disparaging other people's choices.

Voluntarily stopping eating and drinking (VSED) was an imperfect way to conclude his life story, but it was certainly superior to some of the alternatives. He never considered using a violent method because he deeply cared about the potential impact of such a death on his spouse and the other members of the clan. A carefully conceived and well-informed overdose would have served his wishes expeditiously, but it obviously offended some of his family and would have had disastrous consequences if it "failed."

Dan wanted to make a political statement through his death and hoped to accomplish this by candidly chronicling his story. He fully understood that as medical advancements allow for the prolongation of life, discussions about the quality of life and the right to end suffering desperately need to be facilitated. Dan wished medical professionals might discover for themselves the rewards of switching clinical gears from recovery-directed management to instead helping people, like himself, to die well.[8] He was not oblivious that euthanasia, VSED, medical assisted dying, palliative sedation, and lethal overdoses or other forms

---

[7] Nicholas Kristof, "Will Republicans abandon this medical triumph?" Opinion. *The New York Times,* September 20, 2023, accessed September 21, 2023, https://www.nytimes.com/2023/09/20/opinion/republicans-pepfar-aids.html?campaign_id=39&emc=edit_ty_20230921&instance_id=103278&nl=opinion-today&regi_id=63340269&segment_id=145313&te=1&user_id=89534 3099129dcd1f95fa65a5a136796.

[8] G. M. Marcel and Olde Rikkert, "My three-point turn toward personalizing good death in old age," *CMAJ* 195, no. 35 (September 2023): E1184–E1185; DOI: https://doi.org/10.1503/cmaj.230201.

of rational suicide defy traditional legal/ethical normative frameworks.[9] Dan realized that as societies redefine their positions on these practices, they must strike a balance between individual autonomy, medical ethics, and the protection of vulnerable populations. However, he also knew that time was running out, and he needed to make choices for himself.

Dan was optimistic that in the future there will be better options available for people stricken with the different types of dementia. He never dismissed the possibility that medical science will arrive at a cure for these terrible diseases, but Dan correctly perceived it is unlikely to be imminent. He knew that nations like Canada, Switzerland, and Belgium currently offer assisted dying to people who have dementias and still retain capacity, and this option is being actively debated in Australia, New Zealand, and the United States.

Upon reflection, I am confident my mentors would have agreed that Dan achieved a good death. How he died was consistent with how he lived, and he boldly insisted upon having "the type of death one would choose if there were a choice." There are limits to the extent any of us can control how and when we die, but Dan came reasonably close to attaining a better outcome than what he would have experienced if he had passively accepted dementia's otherwise preordained course.

Yes, I think it was a good death.

*****

During my preparatory and background research into *Winter's End*, I discovered numerous other individuals in addition to Dan and Cody Sontage who had dementing illnesses and chose to accelerate their deaths. Prominent among them is Sandra Bem, but they also include Hugo Clause, Janet Adkins, Cheryl Hiebert, Gayle Garlock, Annie Zwijnenberg, Brian Ameche, John Strong Macauley Smith, Ruth Oppenheim, Wayne Briese, Cheryl Hauser, and John L'Heureux.

I have also read several excellent recent bestsellers that explore this theme, including Amy Bloom's memoir in which she movingly describes the assisted death of her husband at a clinic in Switzerland,[10] Dr. Sandeep Jauhar's record of his family's disagreements,[11] and Wendy Mitchell's tender, autobiographical

---

[9] Isha Dhinsna, "Suicide in dementia," in *Dementia Care: Issues, Responses and International Perspectives*, ed. Mala Kapur Shankardass (Singapore: Springer, 2021), 13.

[10] Elisabeth Egan, "When her husband said he wanted to die, Amy Bloom listened," *The New York Times*, accessed January 26, 2023, https://www.nytimes.com/2022/03/01/books/review-in-love-memoir-amy-bloom.html.

[11] Sandeep Jauhar, *My Father's Brain: Life in the Shadow of Alzheimer's* (New York: Farrar, Straus and Giroux, 2023).

account.[12] The latter is the third book written in quick succession by a U.K. native (with the help of a co-writer) who was diagnosed with young-onset vascular dementia and Alzheimer's. This will be her last, and she emphasizes her wish to accelerate dying, along with her frustration over the lack of a medical assistance in dying (MAiD) statute in Great Britain.[13]

Mitchell writes: "If only the medical system offered me an escape route, though; if only those of us who are tired—so tired—could choose instead to rest finally. Not all of us with chronic, progressive or terminal illnesses, but those of us who would prefer to avoid the later stages, those of us who would like to plan the end of life like we have planned every other part of our lives, those of us who would like to say goodbye while we still can, those of us who would like the right to consider assisted dying."

She continues, "The only thing we have no choice in whatsoever is when we are born, but everything else should come down to personal choice, and that includes death. It doesn't seem right that it's still frowned upon or illegal for us to choose when we've had enough, particularly when we've exhausted all the support there is out there for us."

The actress Julianne Moore consulted Wendy Mitchell while preparing for her Oscar winning role in *Still Alice*. At the film's London premiere, Moore thanked her and expressed an insight that also illuminates Dan's experience of the disease. "One of the things I found is that people often simply feel lost," she told the assembled reporters. "Alzheimer's is more akin to an ongoing panic attack where suddenly nothing has any reference."[14]

Dan would have rejoiced at discovering another kindred spirit, like Wendy Mitchell. He would also have been pleased to learn about Gillian Bennett, 85, who ended her Alzheimer's disease with an overdose.[15] The following is an excerpt from the four-page letter Bennett requested that her family post online following her demise.[16]

[12] Wendy Mitchell, *One Last Thing: How to Live with the End in Mind* (London: Bloomsbury Publishing, 2023).

[13] Robert Booth, "Two-thirds of Britons support legalising assisted dying, poll shows," *The Guardian*, accessed August 30, 2023, https://www.theguardian.com/society/2023/aug/28/two-thirds-of-britons-support-legalising-assisted-dying-poll-shows.

[14] Tom Seymour, "Still Alice is 'shockingly accurate': People living with dementia give their verdict," The Guardian. accessed October 7, 2023, https://www.theguardian.com/film/2015/feb/10/still-alice-alzheimers-accurate-dementia-sufferers-verdict.

[15] Cohen, *A Dignified Ending*, 70–73.

[16] Gillian Bennett, "Goodbye & good luck!" Dead at Noon, accessed July 2, 2023, http://deadatnoon.com/index.html.

I will take my life today around noon. It is time. Dementia is taking its toll and I have nearly lost myself. I have nearly lost me.

There comes a time . . . when one is no longer competent to guide one's own affairs. I want out before the day when I can no longer assess my situation or take action to bring my life to an end.

Dementia gives no quarter and admits no bargaining. . . . Ever so gradually at first, much faster now, I am turning into a vegetable . . . .

Understand that I am giving up nothing that I want by committing suicide. All I lose is an indefinite number of years of being a vegetable in a hospital setting, eating up the country's money but having not the faintest idea of who I am.

Each of us is born uniquely and dies uniquely. I think of dying as a final adventure with a predictably abrupt end. I know when it's time to leave and I do not find it scary.

Every day I lose bits of myself, and it's obvious that I am heading towards the state that all dementia patients eventually get to: not knowing who I am and requiring full-time care. I know as I write these words that within six months or nine months or twelve months, I, Gillian, will no longer be here. What is to be done with my carcass? It will be physically alive but there will be no one inside . . . .

If my cat were failing in the way that I am, I would mix some sleeping medication in with top-quality ground beef, and when she fell asleep, carry her lovingly to the garden and do the rest. Who wants to die surrounded by strangers, no matter how excellent their care and competence?

Today, now, I go cheerfully and so thankfully into that good night. [My husband] Jonathan, the courageous, the faithful, the true and the gentle, surrounds me with company. I need no more.

It is almost noon.

Gillian Bennett's Website is called deadatnoon.com. Upon reading this section of the manuscript, bioethicist David N. Hoffman wrote me (June 24, 2023, email): "The first spoon of ice cream is divine, the hundredth perhaps not desirable at all. They are both composed of the same ingredients, but we necessarily experience them very differently. So, it is with life."

Ahhh, so it is with life.

*****

AFTERWORD

Almost exactly two years after Dan's death, Cody Sontag, 71, quietly died.[1] She was a psychotherapist, a birder, an avowedly generous soul who did international rescue work in war-torn Bosnia and Croatia, as well as a regular volunteer in the Mexican village where she wintered.

I reached out to her widow, Judith Roth, who replied (February 8, 2024, email) that "Cody and I both held the vision of wanting to expand choices of dying for people with dementia or Alzheimer's. We openly shared her decision and process with others in the hopes that the vision of choice could become a reality. Cody was clear, she did not want to follow the path of progressive dementia. She empowered herself by making another choice."

Cody was able to make use of a new option that hadn't been available to Dan. She started with voluntarily stopping eating and drinking (VSED), but not as an end in itself. Instead, it became a "bridge" for her to then qualify and make use of MAiD.[2]

In the United States, the consensus has been that people who have dementias are ineligible to receive MAiD for three reasons: they must be able to self-administer the lethal medication *and* retain capacity to make the decision *and* be terminally ill. Dan and most other individuals in the early to middle stage of these diseases are able to generally fulfill the first two requirements but not the last.

However, since Dan died, legal amendments in four US jurisdictions with previously enacted MAiD statutes have shortened or eliminated their required

---

[1] "Cody Jo Ellen Christine Wahto Sontag," *Anchorage Daily News*, Accessed February 12, 2024, https://obituaries.adn.com/adportal/listingView.html?id=5860Please

[2] Thaddeus Mason Pope, and Lisa Brodoff, "Medical aid in dying to avoid late-stage dementia," *Journal of the American Geriatric Society.* 2024; 1–7. doi:10.1111/jgs.18785. https://onlinelibrary.wiley.com/share/author/E5CBVJSZP22YHZNPFRVX?target=10.1111/jgs.18785

waiting periods between determining eligibility and receiving a lethal prescription. This potentially means that people with dementing illnesses may now qualify as having a terminal condition if they begin the process of VSED and exhibit symptoms consistent with dehydration.

Years before, Cody watched her father slowly die from a protracted dementia. Later when she was diagnosed with mild cognitive impairment (MCI) and Alzheimer's disease, Cody conferred with End of Life Choices Oregon volunteer Linda Jensen (February 11, 2024, email), and hospice & palliative medicine specialist Dr. George Drasin. The latter had previously employed this method with another patient suffering from dementia (February 13, 2024, email).

Cody and Judith discussed his novel approach with their loved ones so that everyone would fully understand their decision and support it. The two women were hopeful that by fully disclosing the plan and airing any objections, no one would interfere with Cody's choice of dying.

One year after her cognitive impairment was diagnosed, Cody began with the active involvement of her medical team a reduced calorie diet as a preliminary step of VSED. She was accepted to hospice, and several days later she began full-fledged VSED—completely refraining from ingesting food or fluids. Shortly thereafter, she was evaluated by Dr. Drasin, who determined that she now qualified for MAiD. This was confirmed by a telemedicine consultation with a second physician, and the waiting period was waived. Cody received her lethal prescription, and she ingested the medication two days later. Cody died at home in the presence of her spouse and closest friends.

Opponents of MAiD have reacted predictably to this methodology and consider it to be a "loophole."[3] From their perspective, "There are never enough assisted suicides for the euthanasia movement."

Judith Roth strongly disagrees, as she explained to me, "Cody's experience was uplifting and transformative for us all. And as a result, my grief is nothing like the expected or usual grief."

It remains to be seen whether clinical guidelines are developed for this option, but it leaves me optimistic that legislators will tackle the issue and make assisted dying more available for people who have dementias.

[3] Wesley J. Smith, "Self-starvation to qualify for assisted suicide," *National Review*, February 7, 2024, accessed February 12, 2024, https://www.nationalreview.com/corner/self-starvation-to-qualify-for-assisted-suicide/

CONTRIBUTORS

Sid Adelman, Dementia support group facilitator, Los Angeles

Jacob M. Appel, MD, JD, MPH, Associate Professor of Psychiatry and Medical Education at the Icahn School of Medicine at Mount Sinai

Michael T. Bailin, MD, Associate Professor of Anesthesiology, University of Massachusetts Chan Medical School-Baystate, Chairman Emeritus, Department of Anesthesiology, Baystate Medical Center

Margaret P. Battin, PhD, MFA, Distinguished Professor of Philosophy and Medical Ethics at the University of Utah Medical School

Jan Bernheim, MD, PhD, Professor of Medicine and Medical Ethics, Vrije Universiteit Brussel Faculty of Medicine, Belgium, and co-founder of the International Society of Quality of Life and the first palliative care unit on the European continent

Joan Berzoff, EdD, Professor Emerita at Smith College School for Social Work

Samuel Blouin, PhD in sociology from the Université de Montréal and the Université de Lausanne

Stephen J. Bonasera, MD, PhD, Medical Director of Baystate Medical Center's Memory Assessment and Care Clinic, and Chief, Division of Geriatrics and Palliative Care

William S. Breitbart, MD, Chairman and the Jimmie C. Holland Chair in Psychiatric Oncology, Department of Psychiatry & Behavioral Sciences, Memorial Sloan Kettering Cancer Center

Maura J Brennan, MD, Professor, Department of Medicine at University of Massachusetts Chan Medical School-Baystate

Colin Brewer, MD, retired psychiatrist and board member of My Death, My Decision.

Sandy Buchman, MD, Professor, Division of Palliative Care, University of Toronto, and President, The Canadian Medical Association

Booker Bush, MD, Primary Care Medicine, Baystate Medical Center

Harvey Chochinov, MD, PhD, Distinguished Professor of Psychiatry at the University of Manitoba, and Senior Scientist with CancerCare Manitoba Research Institute

LaVera Crawley, MD, MPH, OFS, CommonSpirit Health System, VP Pastoral and Spiritual Care, San Francisco

Dena S. Davis, JD, PhD, Professor Emerita at Cleveland-Marshall College of Law, and Endowed Presidential Chair in Health (Humanities & Social Sciences) at Lehigh University

Peter A. DePergola II, PhD, MTS, Chief Ethics Officer & Senior Director, Clinical and Organizational Ethics, UMass Chan Medical School-Baystate, and Shaughness Family Chair & Associate Professor of Bioethics and Medical Humanities, Elms College

David Donovan, PhD, Psychologist/Psychoanalyst, Kansas City

Jocelyn Grant Downie OC, FRSC is the James S. Palmer Chair in Public Policy and Law at Schulich School of Law, Canada

Alfonso Fasano, MD, Professor of Neurology at the University of Toronto, Investigator at Krembil Brain Institute, Toronto

Joseph J. Fins, MD, Chief of the Division of Medical Ethics and E. William Davis, Jr., M.D. Professor of Medical Ethics at Weill Cornell Medical College

Brent P. Forester MD, MSc, Dr. Frances S. Arkin Chair of Psychiatry, Tufts University School of Medicine, Professor, Department of Psychiatry

Catherine Frazee, Professor Emerita in the School of Disability Studies at Toronto Metropolitan University, and formerly the Chief Commissioner of the Ontario Human Rights Commission

Ruth von Fuchs, Right to Die Society of Canada activist

Michael Germain, MD, Professor of Medicine, University of Massachusetts-Chan Medical School

Kare Daschiff Gilovich, LCSW, private practitioner

Faye Girsh, EdD, Founder, Hemlock Society of San Diego

Peter Gowin, PhD, Phd, Geschaftsfuher Austria Right to Die Society

Stefanie Green, MD, co-founder and Past President of the Canadian Association of MAID Assessors and Providers, and author of This is Assisted Dying

David R. Grube, MD, National Medical Director of Compassion & Choices (2015-2022), retired Family Physician

Janet Hager, BS in PT, Founding Director and Treasurer of A Better Exit and Treasurer of Hemlock Society of San Diego

Sally Hall, MD, Psychiatrist (retired), Hemlock Society of San Diego (active member)

Robin Maranz Henig, journalist, and author of New York Times Magazine piece on Sandra Bem

Edward Hirsch, poet, and President of John Simon Guggenheim Memorial Foundation

David N. Hoffman, JD, Assistant Professor in Bioethics at Columbia University, School of Professional Studies, and Clinical Assistant Professor in Bioethics at Albert Einstein College of Medicine

Robert K. Horowitz, MD, Gosnell Distinguished Professor in Palliative Care and Chief of Palliative Care Division at the University of Rochester School of Medicine and Dentistry

Rob Jonquière, MD, Executive Director of the World Federation of Right to Die Societies, and former CEO of The Dutch Association for a Voluntary End of Life

Anahid Kabasakalian, MD, MA, Medical Director, IDD/MH Specialty Unit, Kings County Hospital, Brooklyn

Sarah J. Kiskadden-Bechtel, MBe, Program Director, The Completed Life Initiative; Associate Faculty in the Masters of Bioethics program at Columbia University

Benzi M. Kluger, MD, Professor of Neurology and Medicine and Director of the Palliative Care Research Center and Neuropalliative Care Service at the University of Rochester School of Medicine and Dentistry

Mark S. Komrad, MD, psychiatrist and medical ethicist on faculty at Johns Hopkins, University of Maryland. and Tulane

Tara Lagu, MD, Professor of Medicine, Director, Institute for Public Health and Medicine at Northwestern Medicine

Janis Landis, Past-President, Final Exit Network

Barbara Coombs Lee, PA, FNP, JD, President Emerita of Compassion & Choices

Drew and Pauline Lewis, neighbors

Madeline Li, MD, PhD, Associate Professor in the Department of Psychiatry, University of Toronto, and a Clinician Scientist in the Department of Supportive Care, Princess Margaret Cancer Centre

Paul Lippmann, MD, retired training psychoanalyst at Austen Riggs, retired Associate Professor of psychology at Columbia University and the University of Massachusetts, Amherst

Laurie Loisel, Director of Communication & Outreach, Northwestern District Attorney's Office

Stephen Luippold, APRN, psychiatric nurse practitioner

Sylvan Luley, team member of DIGNITAS, Switzerland

Joanne Lynn, MD, MS, MA, is a geriatrician, palliative care authority, and Eldercare Consultant/Advocate

Zachary Macchi, MD, Assistant Professor, Behavioral Neurology & Neuropalliative Care Sections, Department of Neurology, University of Colorado Anschutz Medical Campus

Shannon Mazur, DO, MA, Assistant Professor of Psychiatry, Yale School of Medicine, and Chair of Special Interest Group in Bioethics at the Academy of Consultation-Liaison Psychiatry

Diane Meier, MD, Professor of Geriatrics and Palliative Medicine and Catherine Gaisman Professor of Medical Ethics at the Icahn School of Medicine at Mount Sinai Hospital, Director Emerita and Strategic Medical Advisor of the Center to Advance Palliative Care

Paul T. Menzel, PhD, Professor of Philosophy Emeritus, Pacific Lutheran University, and co-editor of *Voluntarily Stopping Eating and Drinking* (OUP, 2022)

David Meyers, MD, Acting Director for the Agency for Healthcare Research and Quality, which is part of the US Department of Health and Human Services, who spoke to me as a private citizen dealing with a glioblastoma. He was a family practice physician

Kenji Miyamoto, MD, PhD, Professor Emeritus, Hokkaido University and Honorary President, Hokkaido Chuo Rosai Hospital

Reiko Miyamoto, MD, Director of Medical Center for Dementia Diseases, Ebetsu Suzuran Hospital, Director of the Hokkaido Branch of Japan Society for Dying with Dignity

Elizabeth A. Morrison, MD, Forensic Psychiatrist, Chevy Chase

R. Sean Morrison, MD, Ellen and Howard C. Katz Professor and Chair for the Brookdale Department of Geriatrics and Palliative Medicine at Mount Sinai

Alvin H. Moss, MD, Professor of Nephrology, *West Virginia University School of Medicine*, and Director of the Center for Health Ethics & Law

Georges Naasan, MD, Associate Professor of Neurology at Mount Sinai Hospital, Icahn School of Medicine, New York, and Medical Director for the division of Behavioral Neurology and Neuropsychiatry

Philip Nitschke, MD, Founder of Exit International, Switzerland

Chantal Perrot, MD, primary care physician, and a MAID assessor and provider, Canada

Thaddeus Mason Pope, JD, PhD, Professor of Law at Mitchell Hamline School of Law in Saint Paul, Minnesota, and editor of Voluntarily Stopping Eating and Drinking (OUP, 2022)

Tia Powell, MD, Professor, Department of Epidemiology & Population Health and Department of Psychiatry and Behavioral Sciences at the Albert Einstein College of Medicine, Bronx, New York, and Dr. Shoshanah Trachtenberg Frackman Faculty Scholar in Biomedical Ethics

Tim Quill, MD, Professor Emeritus of Medicine, Psychiatry, Medical Humanities, and Nursing at the University of Rochester School of Medicine, past president of American Academy of Hospice and Palliative Medicine, and editor of Voluntarily Stopping Eating and Drinking (OUP)

Rob Rivas, JD, Attorney for Final Exit Network

Gary Rodin, MD. Professor of Psychiatry and Director, Global Institute of Psychosocial Oncology, Palliative Care and End-of-Life -Care (GIPPEC), Princess Margaret Cancer Centre, University of Toronto

James R. Rundell, M.D., Professor of Psychiatry, Uniformed Services University of the Health Sciences School of Medicine, Bethesda MD

Peg Sandeen, PhD, MSW, Chief Executive Officer of Death with Dignity, and Adjunct Professor of Social Work at Columbia University

Jerald Sanders, MD, Medical Director Whidbey Health Hospice, Coupeville, WA

Jane C. Sargent, MD, (deceased) Professor of Neurology, University of Massachusetts Chen School of Medicine

Timothy Schmutte, PsyD, Assistant Professor, Yale University School of Medicine, Department of Psychiatry, Yale Program for Recovery and Community and Health

Judith K. Schwarz, PhD, RN, Clinical Director of End of Life Choices New York, and co-editor of Voluntarily Stopping Eating and Drinking (OUP, 2022)

Lonny Shavelson, MD, Chair, American Clinicians Academy on Medical Aid in Dying

Charles L. Sprung, MD, Professor & Director Emeritus of the General ICU at Hadassah Hebrew University Medical Center in Jerusalem, Israel

Susan Stefan, JD, author of *Rational Suicide, Irrational Laws: Examining Current Approaches to Suicide in Policy and Law* (Oxford University Press, 2016)

Maurice Steinberg, MD, formerly Clinical Professor in Psychiatry, Albert Einstein College of Medicine, and the Zucker School of Medicine

Donna E. Stewart, CM, MD, FRCPC, Emerita Lillian Love Chair or Women's Health at University Health Network, University Professor at University of Toronto, Senior Scientist at Toronto General Hospital Research Institute

Steven Stingley, brother-in-law

Thomas Strouse, MD, Professor of Clinical Psychiatry and the Maddie Katz Endowed Chair in Palliative Care Research and Education, UCLA

Daniel Sulmasy, MD, PhD, André Hellegers Professor of Biomedical Ethics, Departments of Medicine and Philosophy, Director, Kennedy Institute of Ethics, Georgetown University

Rebecca Thoman, MD, Compassion & Choices, Doctors for Dignity Program Director

Beverley Thorn, PhD, retired chair of Clinical Health Psychology at the University of Alabama

Sally Thorne, RN, PhD, School of Nursing, Principal Research Chair in Palliative and End-of-Life Care, University of British Columbia

Konia Trouton, MD, MPH, FCFP, Clinical Professor, Department of Family Medicine at University of British Columbia, MD. Board President for the Canadian Association of MAiD Assessors and Providers

James A. Tulsky, MD, Professor of Medicine, Harvard Medical School, Poorvu Jaffe Chair, Department of Psychosocial Oncology and Palliative Care, Dana-Farber Cancer Institute, and Chief, Division of Palliative Medicine, Medicine, Brigham and Women's Hospital

Tom Tuxill, MD (deceased), Chair, Medical Evaluation Committee and Senior Guide of Final Exit Network

Bea Verbeeck, MD, psychiatrist, Medical Director of Levenslust (Joy of Living), Belgium

Eric Walsh, MD, Emeritus Professor of Family Medicine and Emeritus Professor of Internal Medicine, Oregon Health and Science University, Portland

Ed Weiss, MD, General Practitioner and MAID provider, Ontario

Ellen Wiebe, MD, Clinical Professor in the Department of Family Practice at the University of British Columbia

Els van Wijngaarden, PhD, Associate Professor in Contemporary Meanings of Ageing and Dying, Radboud University Medical Center, Department of Anesthesiology, Pain and Palliative Medicine

Jack Winter, Dan's son

Wynne Winter, Dan's ex-wife

Stuart J. Youngner, MD, Professor Emeritus of Bioethics, Department of Bioethics, Case Western Reserve University, Cleveland

Jeffrey A. Zesiger, MD, Hospice and Palliative Medicine Practitioner, Medical Director, Hospice of the Fisher Home, Amherst, MA

ACKNOWLEDGMENTS

This book is based on 9 months of audiotaped interviews with Dan Winter and John David Forsgren in 2020–2021, as well as subsequent interviews with the latter that took place over a 3-year period following Dan's death. The transcribed interview material before Dan died runs well over 650 single-spaced pages and 325,000 words; it was condensed and edited for clarity.

Upon deciding to write a book about thoughtfully ending one's life if diagnosed with a dementia, I read voraciously about the subject and interviewed many dozens of authorities from North America and Western Europe. I was fortunate in already having contacts within the leadership of the Hemlock Society of San Diego, the World Federation of Right-to-Die Societies, Compassion and Care, the American Clinicians Academy on Medical Aid in Dying and a variety of other organizations. I also reached out to numerous individuals and organizations pledged to oppose death-accelerating practices. All of them contributed to my understanding, and I am exceedingly grateful.

My son, Jake, requested that I complete this writing project as soon as possible. "Dad," he said, "you don't have a dementia, and you're spending way too much time thinking about this subject. Please go and start writing another book." All I can say is, "Jake, I hope you're correct, but I still want to prepare for the distinct possibility that you're wrong."

My son, Zeke, has testified with me on behalf of Maryland's proposed death-with-dignity law (which has yet to be passed), and we will hopefully do it again this year. However, he (and Jake) made it clear they are not eager to directly assist me in ending my life—although they won't throw up insurmountable barriers. We'll see what happens, if or when we reach that point.

My wife, the social work professor, Joan Berzoff, offered more than a few critiques of this book, including the pointed question, "Does the world need yet another white, male, American protagonist?" Maybe or maybe not, but I certainly hope that Dan Winter's story has resonance that goes well beyond his demographics.

It is important to emphatically state that Joan not only tolerated the time and passion I expended on this book, but it was her endless encouragement that allowed me to keep writing throughout the pandemic and into my new phase of my life as a retired academic physician. I could not have emotionally endured this project without regularly telling her what I was encountering. None of us knows with certainty what lies ahead, but she is my anchor.

Science writer Seth Shulman is my cheerleader, critic, neighbor, guru, and friend. He is also incredibly self-effacing and modest about his contributions, but they entirely informed the book. Without his wisdom and encouragement, I would have been hopelessly lost with this and each of my previous literary endeavors.

I have listed about one hundred people who contributed. Many of them read and commented on excerpts from the manuscript through interviews and email exchanges. Some of their additional observations are incorporated into future explanatory articles and online pieces to further explore this subject. These authorities provided both an American and a global perspective of the subject, which allowed me to feel intellectually grounded during my writing. I wanted to especially cite a few of them, including Dr. Tim Quill, the late Dr. Jane Sargent (who I will always recall as having been my favorite neurologist), Fay Girsh, Derek Humphry, Peg Sandeen, Dr. Philip Nitschke, Paul Mentzel, and Dr. Madeline Li.

There are a large number of friends, colleagues, and new acquaintances who sit on the opposite side of the aisle from me when it comes to assisted dying, and their involvement was crucial in lending balance to this book. They include but are not limited to Dr. Sean Morrison, Dr. Joseph Fins, Professor Catherine Frazee, Dr. William Breitbart, and Dr. Harvey Chochinov.

Interviews were conducted with Dan's psychologist, Dr. David Donovan, and his neighbors, Pauline and Drew Lewis. In addition, Daryl Bem, Robin Marantz Henig, and several of Sandy Bem's circle of friends were exceedingly kind in answering my many questions about her life. I spoke several times with Dr. Eric Walsh and hope he's still consulting when I require the help of a wise hospice and palliative medicine physician. The wonderfully acerbic Judith Schwarz and the ageless rebel Dr. Joanne Lynn both generously offered their insights, as well as made me laugh. I discovered the story of Cody Sontag as the manuscript was being proofed, and I'd like to express my thanks to Judith Ross, Linda Jensen, Lisa Brodoff, and Dr. George Drasin; Fabian Shalini was the Production Editor who helped me through this obstacle.

I must acknowledge my artistic and intellectual debt to a number of books and films beginning with Katie Engelhart's *The Inevitable* (St. Martin's Press, 2021), Timothy E. Quill, et al.'s *Voluntarily Stopping Eating and Drinking* (Oxford University Press, 2021), and Lisa Genova's *Still Alice* (Simon & Schuster, 2007). But others include Amy Bloom's *In Love: A Memoir of Love and Loss* (Random House, 2022), Sandeep Jauhar's *My Father's Brain: Life in the Shadow of Alzheimer's* (Farrar, Straus, and Giroux, 2023), Barbara Coombs Lee's *Finish Strong* (CompassionandChoices.org, 2021), Tracy Kidder's *Mountains Beyond Mountains* (Penguin Random House, 2003), Mitch Albom's *Tuesdays with Morrie* (Doubleday, 1997), Wendy Mitchell's *One Last Thing: How to Live with the End in Mind* (Bloomsbury, 2023), as well as Irwin and Marilyn Yalom's dying collaboration in *A Matter of Death and Life* (Redwood Press, 2021). The films *Supernova* (2021), starring Stanley Tucci and Colin Firth, and *The Father* (2020), featuring Anthony Hopkins, are required viewing!

Nowadays, it is incredibly unfashionable to give Sigmund Freud credit for anything, but his life and the way he died have long inspired me. I was enthralled by his lengthy case histories—be they the stories of the Wolf Man, the Rat Man, and especially Anna O—while my time spent studying with his daughter, Anna Freud, remains the intellectual high-water mark of my medical training.

I would like to thank my enthusiastic editor, Marta Moldvai, and her staff from Oxford University Press for helping bring *Winter's End* into the world. Marta was absolutely the most supportive, brightest, and sensible editor that I've ever encountered. Plus, she is obviously a wonderful mother and human being. Her efforts allowed the book to become as true to life as possible while simultaneously striving to approach this complex subject in a scholarly manner.

Several friends were meaningful sounding boards who provided encouragement throughout this process, including Drs. Jeff Zesiger, J. Michael Bostwick, Booker Bush, Michael Bailin, and Jay Holtzman. I'm grateful to nurses Rorry Zahourek and Stephen Luippold, as well as my Sherlock Holmes psychologist, Dr. Jaine Darwin.

I am indebted to those contributors who reviewed and edited relevant sections of the manuscript or referred me to their colleagues, including neurologists Drs. Alfonso Fasano, Bradford C. Dickerson, and Benzi Kluger. Professor Jocelyn Downie helped me to better navigate the Canadian laws, while Dr. Stefanie Green explained how they are being applied. Dr. James Rundell aided me to be more sensitive to social issues, while Drs. Rob Jonquiere and Jan Bernheim provided essential European perspectives and contacts. Drs. Ben Liptzin (my former chairman at Baystate Medical Center) and Maurice Steinberg (my first attending psychiatrist from residency training days) offered critical readings of the entire manuscript.

I would like to express my appreciation to Steve Stingley, who allowed me to see the manuscript he wrote about his brother-in-law. It contains tender anecdotes gleaned from the memories of Dan, his sister, and other family members.

Wynne Winter and Jack Winter graciously participated in what had to have been painful interviews about Dan; both made it clear to me they were speaking only for themselves and not the extended family. I want them and the entire Winter clan—siblings, children, spouse, nephews, nieces, and various in-laws— to know how much I tried to be respectful of the story's complexity and their obvious affection for Dan. I sincerely apologize if I misinterpreted any of the events or hurt anyone's feelings.

> O, but they say the tongues of dying men
> Enforce attention like deep harmony.
> Where words are scarce, they are seldom spent in
> vain,
> For they breathe truth that breathe their words in pain.
>
> —*Richard II*, Act 2, Scene 1, William Shakespeare

John and Dan provided me with an extraordinary opportunity to take a close look at their lives at a time in which most people bolt the door, climb into bed, and pull the covers over their heads. I lack adequate words (a terrible thing for an author to confess) to express my gratitude to them. We will always be bound by our dread of Alzheimer's, as well as by the fervent desire to prevent it from assuming total control over our lives, our deaths, and that of others.

INDEX